Glycemic load diet cookbook

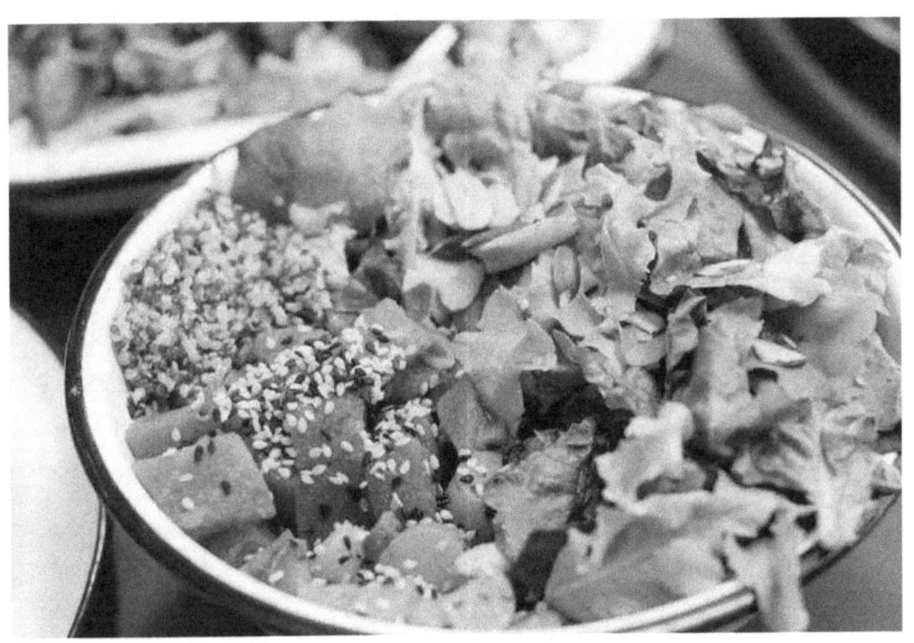

Garry Coleman

Disclaimer
This book is provided for informational purposes only and does not constitute medical, nutritional, or dietary advice. The information contained in this book is based on research and personal experience, and individual results may vary. Readers are encouraged to consult with healthcare professionals and registered dietitians for personalized dietary recommendations and guidance

Contents

Introduction

Once upon a time, in a world where culinary choices danced between taste and health, there existed a magical book – the "Glycemic Load Diet Cookbook and Recipe." It wasn't just a collection of recipes; it was a chronicle of a remarkable journey, a tale of gastronomic exploration veiled in the mystique of glycemic balance. In a quaint village nestled amid rolling hills, there lived an inquisitive chef named Abigail. She possessed an insatiable curiosity for the alchemy of flavors and the science behind nutrition. Her bustling kitchen was a cauldron of creativity, where pots bubbled with tales of taste and health.

One sunny morning, while concocting her culinary marvels, Abigail stumbled upon an ancient parchment filled with secrets untold. It spoke of a forgotten art – the delicate interplay between glycemic loads and the symphony of flavors. With wide-eyed wonder and an eager heart, she embarked on a quest to unlock this enchanting knowledge, unaware of the transformative journey that lay ahead.

Through bustling markets and serene orchards, she sought wisdom from wise sages and seasoned cooks, absorbing every tidbit of knowledge like a parched land drink in the rain. Each encounter unveiled a fragment of the puzzle, painting a vibrant tapestry of low glycemic wonders that could delight both the palate and nourish the soul. As Abigail's quest unfolded, the pages of her cookbook began to breathe with life. Every recipe became a chapter in this odyssey, a testament to the delicate balance of taste and health. She crafted dishes that whispered tales of satiety without sacrifice, where indulgence wasn't a sin but a celebration of nourishment.

With each turn of the page, readers were invited into Abigail's world – a world where breakfasts were a revitalizing symphony, where starters and snacks were tantalizing bites of wholesomeness, and where main courses were a harmony of healthy grains and plant-based wonders. Desserts weren't just a sweet ending but a delightful promise of guilt-free enjoyment. But this book was more than a collection of recipes. It was a narrative woven with threads of inspiration and transformation. It wasn't just about what you ate; it was an invitation to embrace a lifestyle where every meal became an opportunity for a healthier, more vibrant you.

So, dear reader, open this book and embark on Abigail's journey – a journey into the heart of taste, health, and the magic of the glycemic load diet. Let these pages be your guide, and may each recipe be a step toward a more nourished, more fulfilled you. Get ready to indulge in the delight of flavors and the nurturing embrace of a low glycemic world.

Bon appétit and here's to the sweet serenade of health and happiness!

Chapter 1: Understanding Glycemic Load

The food industry is starting to use and discuss the idea of the glycaemic load more and more. The glycaemic index (GI), which compares the impact of an equivalent quantity of pure sugar on blood sugar levels to the effect of a food high in carbohydrates, is a concept that most people are likely familiar with. But the issue with the GI is that it doesn't give a whole picture of the food's ability to raise blood sugar levels. The amount and quality of carbs ingested affect the response of blood sugar. Only the rate at which a carbohydrate becomes sugar is indicated by the GI; it does not tell us how much of a given carbohydrate is present in a dish of food.

Glycemic load, a term closely linked to glycemic index (GI), is a measure of how a certain diet affects blood sugar levels. A food's GI, which ranges from 1 to 100 (100 being the fastest conversion rate), indicates how quickly a food breaks down into glucose. By accounting for both the rate of glucose conversion and the quantity of carbohydrates in a particular meal, GL goes one step further.

How is the glycaemic load calculated?

A food's glycaemic load assigns a number to how much of an impact a certain serving size has on blood sugar levels. It is computed by taking the food's GI value and multiplying it by the quantity of carbohydrates in the dish, then dividing the result by 100. Every GL unit represents the glycaemic impact of one gram of carbohydrates from white bread, with white bread serving as the baseline reference. Using a popular fruit like an apple as an example, the GL is ascertained as follows:

GI of a standard apple = 40
Carbohydrate content of a standard apple = 15
GL = (GI x Carbohydrate content) / 100
= (40 x 15) / 100
= 6

When two foods have the same GI value but Food A has 5% carbs and Food B has 80% carbs, Food B has a higher GL and therefore to be consumed in smaller amounts. Generally speaking, foods high in carbohydrates and poor in fiber have high GI and GL values, while those high in fiber have lower GLs.

Elements that impact the glycaemic load

The GL of a dish is influenced by several factors. Many of them are comparable to those that affect a food product's GI as well. These include the food's starch and sugar content, preparation methods, fat, fiber, and carbohydrate content, as well as the portion size. The rate at which food items are absorbed and digested affects the GI and GL as well.

Typically, the GL of a given food is determined using the ranges listed below:

- Low GL – 10 or less
- Medium GL – 11 to 19
- High GL – 20 or more

The GL per day is defined by applying the following values:

- Low GL – less than 80
- High GL – more than 120

Refined snack foods like chips and sweetened beverages, as well as white rice, are high GL foods. The general rise in blood sugar levels is slower and lower when low-GL foods are consumed.

The benefits of the GL have been established; for individuals with diabetes, in particular, the GL has proven to be a more reflecting and accurate predictor of blood sugar levels. Diabetics can lower their average blood sugar levels and lower their risk of problems like kidney, nerve, and eye damage by following a low-GL diet.

Metabolism and glycaemic load
The GI is not as intricate as the GL. Foods differ in the amount and quality of their carbohydrates (GI values). The GI values of foods with varying carbohydrate densities will be compared.

A baked potato is on the list of foods to avoid or consume less of because of its medium-high GI designation. Watermelon also has a high GI. A 100g portion of watermelon has 5g of carbohydrates, yet a serving of watermelon has a high water content and a low carbohydrate content. The watermelon's GL value is consequently low. The potato's high GI value is attributed to its higher carbohydrate content. Therefore, compared to a dish of potatoes, eating a watermelon has a considerably lower effect on blood sugar levels. Because potatoes are heavy in carbohydrates, their GL is equally high, hence their GI is not deceptive. Conversely, watermelon has a low GL and a high GI level since it has a low percentage of carbs in it.

Glycaemic load and medical problems
The effect of carbohydrate consumption on long-term heart and major artery health was evaluated by examining more than 75,000 middle-aged, healthy women who were included in the Nurses Health Study.

Regardless of whether the women had traditional heart disease risk factors (such as high blood pressure, high cholesterol, smoking, family history, etc.), they discovered that diets with a high GL value were correlated with a likelihood of heart and major artery disease. Additionally, there was a significant correlation with weight; in particular, dietary GL was positively associated with cardiovascular disease in overweight women. The two did not appear to be significantly associated in lean women. 280 postmenopausal women participated in another study that revealed dietary GL was directly correlated with triglycerides and low-density lipoproteins (LDL) and negatively correlated with HDL levels.

Awareness and managing your diabetes requires an understanding of your blood sugar levels and insulin resistance. Reduced insulin production and elevated insulin resistance have been associated with persistently elevated blood sugar levels following meals. Studies conducted on patients have demonstrated that eating a meal with a low glycaemic index or glycaemic load reduces the rise in blood sugar levels. Diets rich in whole grains and total fiber were linked to lower levels of insulin resistance in the Framingham Study. Insulin resistance has been linked to elevated dietary glycaemic load and glycaemic index. It has also been demonstrated that a lower intake of fiber and a higher intake of glycaemic foods are associated with a higher risk of developing the metabolic syndrome.

Reducing the glycemic load of food

Among the strategies for lowering dietary GL are:

- Eat low-GI foods rather than high-GI ones; swap out carbohydrates for protein;
- Aim to have three or more low-GL items with every meal of the day.

Benefits of Glycemic Load

1. Stabilized Blood Sugar Levels: Low glycemic load diets can assist in stabilizing blood sugar levels. Foods with a lower glycemic load cause a slower and steadier rise in blood sugar, preventing rapid spikes and crashes, which is particularly helpful for individuals with diabetes or insulin resistance.

2. Improved Weight Management: This diet aids in weight management by promoting satiety and reducing cravings. Low glycemic load foods tend to keep you fuller for longer periods, preventing overeating and helping in weight maintenance or weight loss efforts.

3. Enhanced Energy Levels: The slow and steady release of glucose from low glycemic load foods can provide sustained energy throughout the day. This can prevent energy slumps and promote a more consistent energy level, aiding in better focus and productivity.

4. Better Heart Health: Adopting a low glycemic load diet may contribute to improved heart health. It can help in reducing the risk factors associated with heart disease, such as lowering cholesterol levels and managing blood pressure.

5. Improved Mood and Cognitive Function: Stable blood sugar levels resulting from a low glycemic load diet can positively impact mood and cognitive function. Avoiding rapid fluctuations in blood sugar can help in maintaining a more stable mood and clearer thinking.

6. Reduced Risk of Chronic Diseases: Studies suggest that a diet based on low glycemic load foods may decrease the risk of developing chronic diseases such as type 2 diabetes, certain cancers, and even some neurological disorders.

Chapter 2: glycemic load rules and weight loss

Adhering to a glycemic load diet involves several principles to help maintain stable blood sugar levels and reap its benefits:

1. Choose Low Glycemic Load Foods: Emphasize foods with a low glycemic load, such as non-starchy vegetables, legumes, whole grains, nuts, seeds, and most fruits (in moderation).

2. Be Mindful of Portion Sizes: While focusing on low glycemic load foods, pay attention to portion sizes. Even healthy foods can impact blood sugar if consumed excessively.

3. Include Protein and Healthy Fats: Combining low glycemic load carbohydrates with protein and healthy fats can further slow down the absorption of glucose, aiding in better blood sugar control.

4. Avoid Refined Carbohydrates: Minimize intake of highly processed and refined carbohydrates like sugary snacks, white bread, and sugary beverages as they tend to have a higher glycemic load.

5. Favor Whole Foods: Opt for whole, unprocessed foods whenever possible. Whole grains, vegetables, and fruits in their natural form usually have a lower glycemic load compared to processed alternatives.

6. Balanced Meal Planning: Structure meals to include a variety of food groups – carbohydrates, proteins, healthy fats, and fiber. This balance helps in controlling blood sugar levels and maintaining satiety.

8. Regular Monitoring: For those with specific health concerns like diabetes, regular monitoring of blood sugar levels can help in understanding how different foods affect their blood glucose.

By following these guidelines, individuals can effectively adhere to a glycemic load diet, promoting better blood sugar management and overall health.

Weight loss

The glycemic load diet can play a significant role in weight loss due to several reasons:

1. Satiety and Reduced Cravings: Foods with a lower glycemic load tend to provide longer-lasting feelings of fullness and satiety. This can help in reducing overall calorie intake as people are less likely to feel hungry between meals, thus aiding in weight loss efforts.

2. Stabilized Blood Sugar Levels: Consuming foods with a lower glycemic load leads to a more gradual rise in blood sugar levels, preventing rapid spikes and crashes. This steadier blood sugar can help control hunger hormones, reducing the likelihood of overeating and snacking on high-calorie foods.

3. Fat Storage Regulation: High-glycemic foods can promote the body's storage of fats, while lower-glycemic foods are less likely to trigger excess fat storage. This aspect may contribute to more efficient weight management.

4. Enhanced Fat Burning: Lower glycemic load foods are often associated with a more stable insulin response. This stability can promote the body's ability to burn stored fat for energy, potentially aiding in weight loss.

5. Better Adherence to Healthy Eating Patterns: The glycemic load diet encourages the consumption of whole, nutrient-dense foods, promoting a healthier eating pattern that can facilitate weight loss and maintenance in the long term.

It's essential to note that while the glycemic load diet can be helpful for weight loss, it's most effective when combined with regular physical activity, portion control, and an overall balanced diet. Individual responses to dietary changes can vary, so personalized adjustments may be necessary to achieve optimal weight loss results.

Glycemic load diet for diabetes control

The glycemic load diet can be beneficial for individuals managing diabetes as it focuses on foods that minimize blood sugar spikes. Here's how this diet can aid in diabetes control:

1. Balancing Blood Sugar Levels

- ***Choosing Low Glycemic Load Foods***: Emphasizing foods with a low glycemic load helps prevent rapid increases in blood sugar levels after meals. This includes non-starchy vegetables, legumes, whole grains, and certain fruits.
- ***Controlling Portion Sizes:*** Monitoring portion sizes of carbohydrate-rich foods, even those with a low glycemic load, is crucial to manage blood sugar levels effectively.

2. Enhancing Insulin Sensitivity
Reducing Insulin Spikes: By opting for foods that produce slower and more controlled increases in blood sugar, the glycemic load

diet can potentially reduce the demand for insulin, aiding in better insulin sensitivity over time.

3. Weight Management

Supporting Weight Control: The diet's focus on whole, nutrient-dense foods and its ability to prevent sharp rises and crashes in blood sugar levels can aid in weight management. Maintaining a healthy weight is important for managing diabetes.

4. Cardiovascular Health:

Improving Heart Health: Following a glycemic load diet might positively impact cardiovascular health by helping control blood sugar levels, which in turn can reduce the risk of heart disease, a common concern for individuals with diabetes.

5. Customization and Monitoring:

Individualized Approach: It's important for individuals with diabetes to tailor the diet based on their specific needs and responses to different foods. Regular monitoring of blood sugar levels is crucial to gauge the impact of the diet on individual glycemic control.

6. Collaboration with Healthcare Providers:

Consulting Healthcare Professionals: It's advisable for individuals with diabetes to work with healthcare providers, such as dietitians or diabetes educators, to develop a personalized glycemic load diet plan that aligns with their specific health needs and medication management.

Overall, the glycemic load diet, when carefully planned and personalized, can be a valuable tool in managing blood sugar levels and supporting overall health for individuals with diabetes. However, it's essential to approach any dietary changes for diabetes control under the guidance of healthcare professionals to ensure safety and efficacy.

Chapter 3: Eating healthy

3.1 Eating low glycemic load and anti-inflammatory foods

Incorporating both low glycemic load and anti-inflammatory foods into your diet can offer numerous health benefits:

Low Glycemic Load Foods

Non-Starchy Vegetables: Such as leafy greens, broccoli, cauliflower, bell peppers, and tomatoes are excellent choices with a low glycemic load. They provide essential nutrients, fiber, and antioxidants without spiking blood sugar levels.

Legumes: Beans, lentils, and chickpeas are rich in fiber and protein while having a low glycemic load. They contribute to stable blood sugar and offer satiety.

Whole Grains: Opt for whole grains like quinoa, barley, brown rice, and oats over refined grains. They have a lower glycemic load and provide more nutrients and fiber.

Anti-Inflammatory Foods

Berries: Blueberries, strawberries, and raspberries are packed with antioxidants and anti-inflammatory compounds that support overall health.

Fatty Fish: Salmon, mackerel, sardines, and trout are high in omega-3 fatty acids, known for their anti-inflammatory properties.

Nuts and Seeds: Almonds, walnuts, flaxseeds, and chia seeds contain healthy fats and antioxidants that help combat inflammation.

Healthy Fats: Olive oil, avocados, and coconut oil offer monounsaturated fats and antioxidants that have anti-inflammatory effects.

Combining Low Glycemic Load and Anti-Inflammatory Foods:

Balanced Meals: Create meals that combine both types of foods. For example, a salad with leafy greens, colorful veggies, beans (low glycemic load), and topped with olive oil (anti-inflammatory).
Snack Options: Enjoy snacks like a handful of nuts with berries or veggies with hummus, combining the benefits of low glycemic load and anti-inflammatory properties.
Whole Food Choices: Opt for whole, unprocessed foods as they often contain both low glycemic load and anti-inflammatory properties naturally.

By combining these two approaches, individuals can not only manage blood sugar levels effectively but also potentially reduce inflammation in the body. This combination supports overall health and may contribute to better management of conditions influenced by both blood sugar levels and inflammation, such as diabetes and certain autoimmune disorders.

3.2 Avoiding high glycemic and inflammatory foods

Avoiding high glycemic and inflammatory foods can significantly benefit overall health and well-being. Here's a guide on foods to minimize or avoid:

High Glycemic Load Foods to Avoid

Refined Grains: White bread, white rice, and most processed cereals tend to have a high glycemic load, causing rapid spikes in blood sugar levels.
Sugary Snacks and Sweets: Candies, pastries, cakes, cookies, and sugary drinks often lead to quick increases in blood sugar.

Processed Foods: Highly processed foods with added sugars, such as fast food items and certain packaged snacks, tend to have a higher glycemic load.

Inflammatory Foods to Minimize

Trans Fats: Avoid or limit foods containing trans fats, such as margarine, fried foods, and many commercially baked goods.
Highly Processed Foods: Foods with additives, preservatives, and artificial ingredients can contribute to inflammation. This includes many packaged snacks, processed meats, and some ready-to-eat meals.
Sugary Beverages: Regular consumption of sugary drinks like soda can promote inflammation in the body.
Excessive Red and Processed Meats: High consumption of red meat and processed meats like sausages and bacon has been associated with increased inflammation.

Strategies to Minimize High Glycemic and Inflammatory Foods:

Read Labels: Check food labels for added sugars, trans fats, and artificial additives. Opt for products with fewer processed ingredients.
Choose Whole Foods: Place a focus on complete, unprocessed foods including fruits, vegetables, whole grains, lean proteins, and healthy fats.
Cook at Home: Prepare meals at home using fresh ingredients to have more control over what goes into your food.
Portion Control: If you choose to consume higher glycemic or inflammatory foods occasionally, practice moderation and portion control.

supporting overall health for individuals with diabetes. However, it's essential to approach any dietary changes for diabetes control under the guidance of healthcare professionals to ensure safety and efficacy.

Chapter 4: Meal guideline

4.1 stocking your kitchen

Stocking your kitchen with low glycemic load foods is essential for maintaining a diet that helps manage blood sugar levels. Here are some tips for stocking your kitchen with these nutritious options:

1. Whole Grains

Options: Choose whole grains like quinoa, brown rice, barley, bulgur, and whole grain pasta. When compared to refined grains, they have a lower glycemic load.

Tip: Store these grains in airtight containers to maintain freshness and ensure they're readily available for meals.

2. Legumes

Varieties: Stock up on lentils, chickpeas, black beans, and kidney beans. They're rich in fiber and have a low glycemic load.

Preparation: Consider having canned or pre-cooked legumes for quick meal preparation. Dried legumes need soaking and cooking but can be stored for longer periods.

3. Fresh Produce

Colorful Vegetables: Include a variety of non-starchy vegetables like spinach, kale, broccoli, bell peppers, zucchini, and tomatoes. They're low in calories and have a low glycemic load.

Fruits: Opt for low glycemic fruits such as berries (blueberries, strawberries), apples, citrus fruits, and cherries. These provide vitamins, fiber, and antioxidants.

Storage: Store fruits and vegetables properly to maintain their freshness and nutritional value. You can freeze some for later use.

4. Healthy Fats

Nuts and Seeds: Have a selection of almonds, walnuts, chia seeds, flaxseeds, and pumpkin seeds. They're sources of healthy fats, protein, and fiber with a low glycemic load.

Oils: Choose olive oil, avocado oil, or coconut oil for cooking or as dressings. They offer healthy fats and are low on the glycemic index.

5. Dairy and Dairy Alternatives

Greek Yogurt: Opt for plain Greek yogurt or unsweetened yogurt with active cultures. It's a protein-rich option with a lower glycemic load compared to flavored yogurts.

Plant-Based Alternatives: Consider almond milk, coconut milk, or oat milk as dairy substitutes. Choose unsweetened varieties to keep the glycemic load lower.

6. Tips for Stocking

Plan Ahead: Create a shopping list based on your meal plans for the week, ensuring you have a variety of low glycemic load options.

Read Labels: Check food labels for added sugars and high glycemic ingredients to make informed choices.

Limit Processed Foods: Minimize processed snacks, sugary beverages, and pre-packaged meals with high glycemic loads.

Storage Organization: Arrange your kitchen so that healthier options are more accessible, encouraging better choices.

Stocking your kitchen with a variety of low glycemic load foods and keeping them readily available helps create a foundation for preparing balanced meals that support blood sugar management and overall health.

4.2 some List of low glycemic load food

1. Non-Starchy Vegetables
- Spinach
- Kale
- Broccoli
- Cauliflower
- Bell Peppers
- Zucchini
- Cabbage
- Brussels Sprouts
- Asparagus
- Green Beans
- Cucumber
- Eggplant

2. Legumes
- Lentils
- Chickpeas
- Black Beans
- Kidney Beans
- Pinto Beans
- Navy Beans
- Split Peas

3. Whole Grains
- Quinoa
- Brown Rice
- Barley
- Bulgur
- Buckwheat
- Oats (steel-cut or rolled)
- Millet

4. Fruits (in moderation)

- Berries (Strawberries, Blueberries, Raspberries)
- Apples
- Pears
- Oranges
- Cherries
- Plums
- Grapefruit
- Kiwi
- Peaches

5. Nuts and Seeds

- Almonds
- Walnuts
- Chia Seeds
- Flaxseeds
- Pumpkin Seeds
- Sunflower Seeds

6. Dairy and Dairy Alternatives

- Greek Yogurt (plain, unsweetened)
- Unsweetened Almond Milk
- Unsweetened Coconut Yogurt
- Cottage Cheese

7. Healthy Fats

- Olive Oil
- Avocado
- Coconut Oil
- Flaxseed Oil

8. Protein Sources
- Skinless Chicken
- Turkey
- Fish (Salmon, Mackerel, Tuna)
- Tofu
- Tempeh

These low glycemic load foods offer a range of nutrients, including fiber, vitamins, minerals, and healthy fats, while minimizing the impact on blood sugar levels. Incorporating these foods into your meals can help maintain more stable energy levels and support overall health, particularly for those aiming to manage blood sugar levels or following a glycemic load-based diet.

4.3. 7 days meal plan

Day 1:

Breakfast: Greek Yogurt Berry Bowl

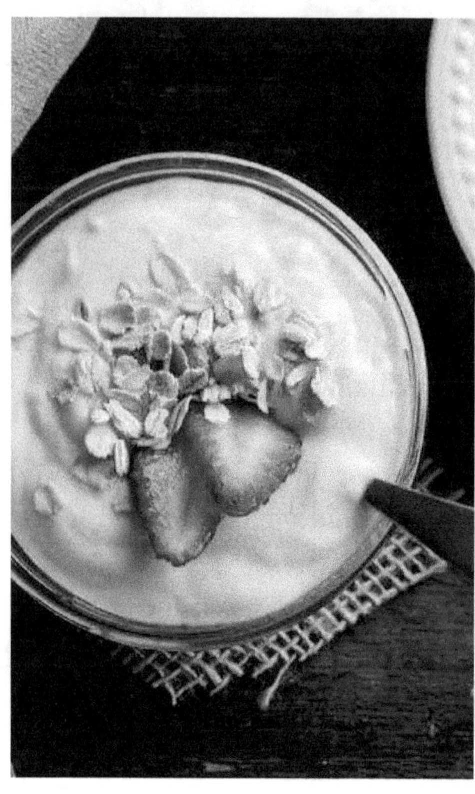

Breakfast: Greek Yogurt Berry Bowl

INGREDIENTS

-1 cup plain Greek yogurt

-½ cup mixed berries (blueberries, strawberries)

-2 tablespoons chopped almonds.

INSTRUCTIONS

Mix Greek yogurt with berries and top with chopped almonds.

NUTRITION INFO:

Fat: 20%, Protein: 35%, Carbs: 45%, Total Calories: ~300

Lunch: Quinoa and Veggie Salad

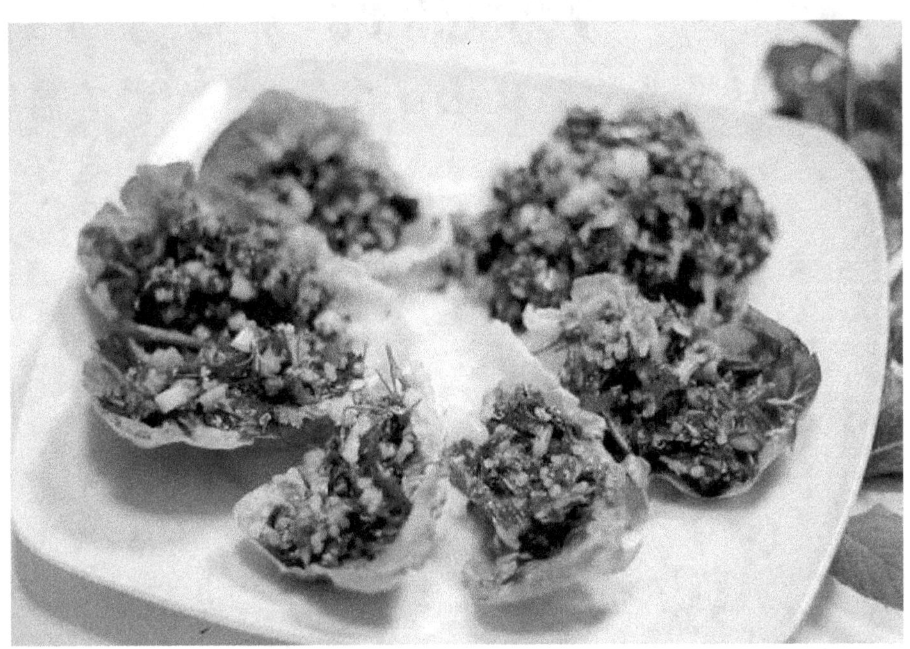

INGREDIENTS

-1 cup cooked quinoa
mixed veggies
(cucumbers
bell peppers
-cherry tomatoes)
-olive oil
-lemon juice
-fresh herbs.

INSTRUCTIONS

1. Combine cooked quinoa with diced veggies

2. dress with olive oil

3. lemon juice

4. and herbs.

NUTRITION INFO:

Fat: 25%, Protein: 15%, Carbs: 60%, Total Calories: ~400

Dinner: Baked Salmon with Steamed Vegetables

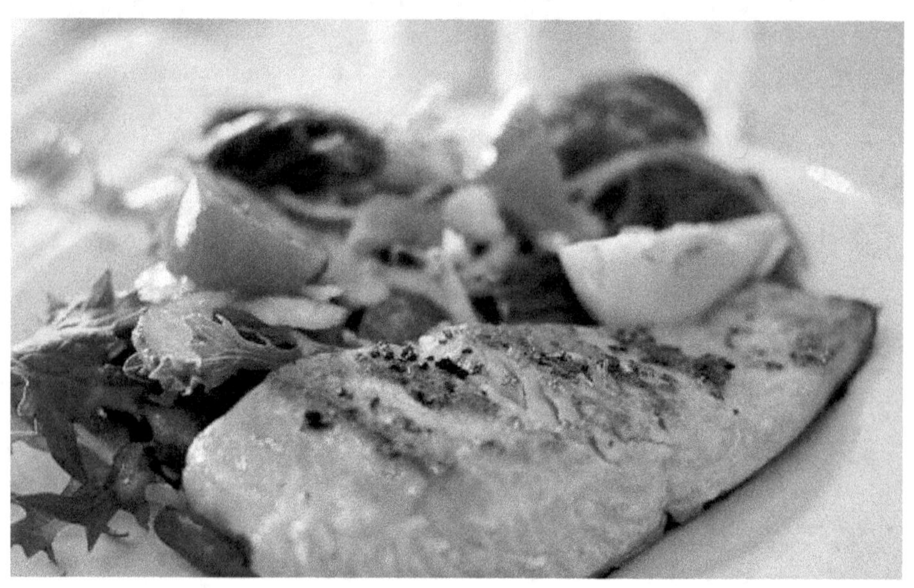

INGREDIENTS

-Salmon filet
-mixed vegetables (broccoli, carrots)
-olive oil
-seasoning.

INSTRUCTIONS

1. Season salmon

2. bake

3. and serve with steamed veggies dressed with a drizzle of olive oil.

NUTRITION INFO:

Fat: 25%, Protein: 15%, Carbs: 60%, Total Calories: ~400

Day 2
Breakfast: Avocado Toast with Poached Egg

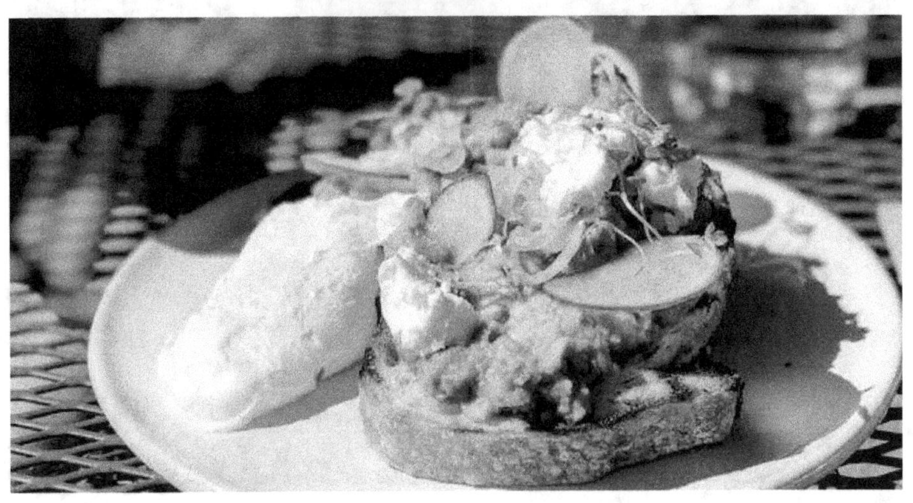

INGREDIENTS

-whole grain bread

 -avocado

-poached egg.

INSTRUCTIONS

1.Toast bread

2. Spread mashed avocado

3. Top with a poached egg.

NUTRITION INFO:

Fat: 40%, Protein: 25%, Carbs: 35%, Total Calories: ~350

Lunch: Quinoa Salad with Chickpeas

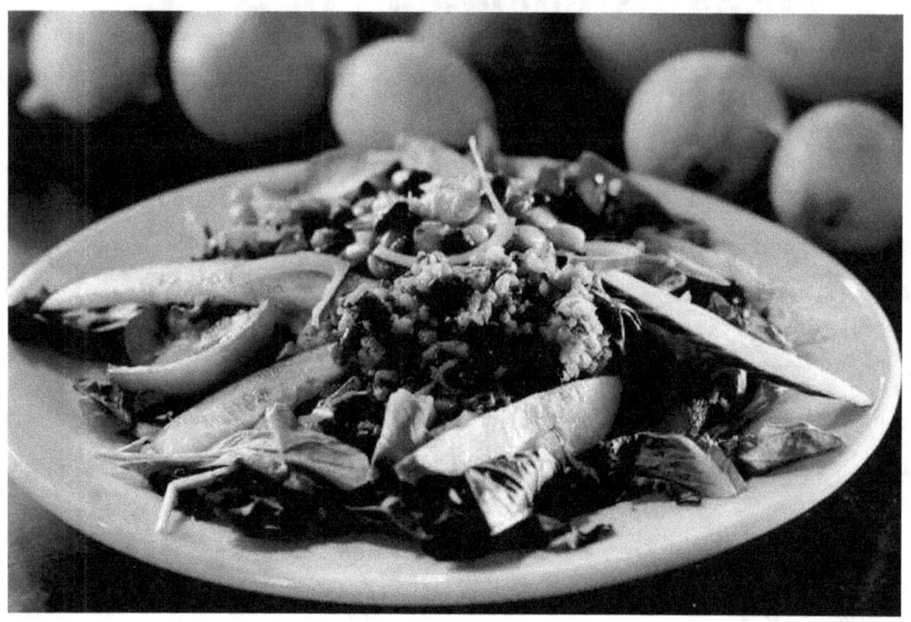

INGREDIENTS

- Cooked quinoa
- chickpeas
- cucumber
- cherry tomatoes
- feta cheese
- olive oil
- lemon juice.

INSTRUCTIONS

1. Mix all ingredients
2. drizzle with olive oil and lemon juice.

NUTRITION INFO:

Fat: 30%, Protein: 20%, Carbs: 50%, Total Calories: ~400

Dinner: Baked Chicken with Steamed Broccoli and Brown Rice

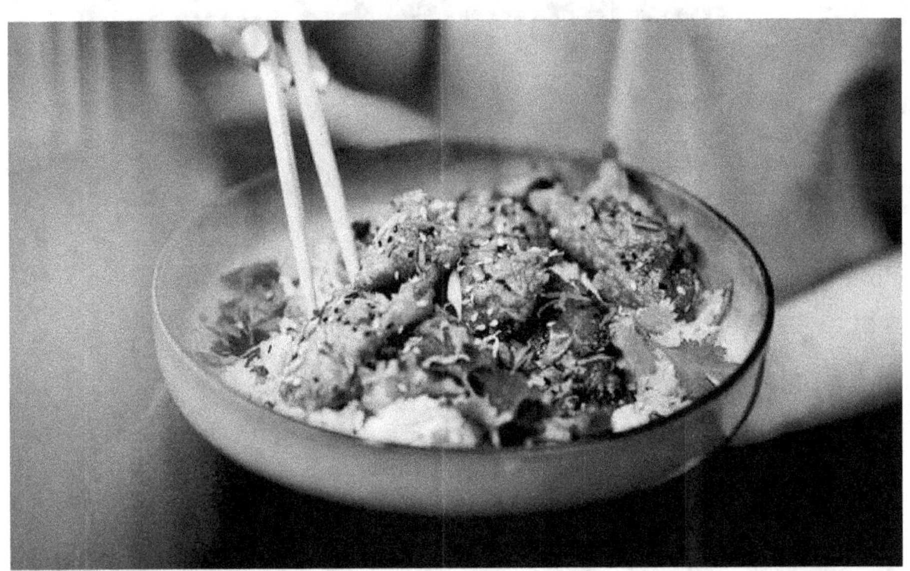

INGREDIENTS

-Chicken breast

-broccoli

-brown rice

-and seasoning.

INSTRUCTIONS

1. Season chicken

2. bake

3. serve with steamed broccoli and brown rice.

NUTRITION INFO:

15%, Protein: 40%, Carbs: 45%, Total Calories: ~450

Day 3
Breakfast: Spinach and Tomato Omelette with Avocado

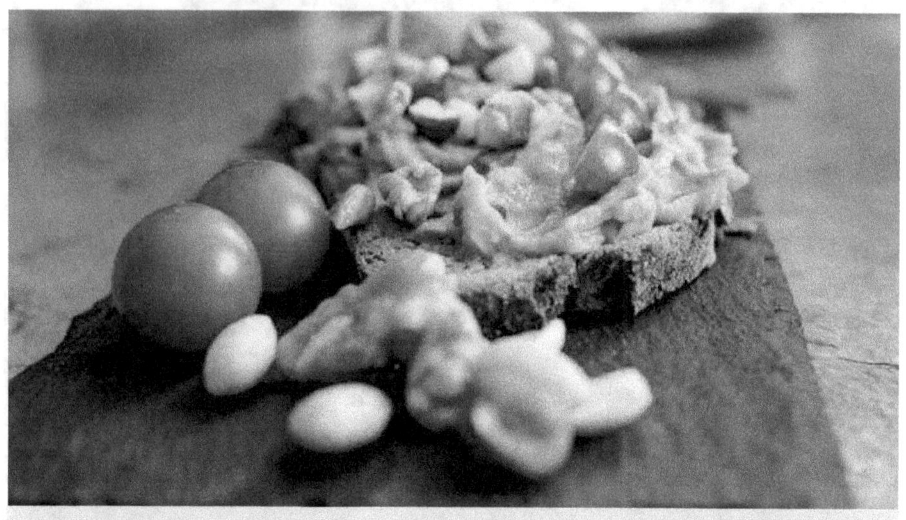

INGREDIENTS

-2 eggs
-1/2 cup spinach
-1/4 cup chopped tomatoes
-1/4 avocado
-1 tablespoon olive oil.

INSTRUCTIONS

1. eggs with spinach and tomatoes
2. Fill an omelet with avocado slices and drizzle with olive oil.

NUTRITION INFO:

35% fat, 25% protein, 40% carbs, 400 calories.

Lunch: Quinoa Salad with Grilled Chicken and Vegetable

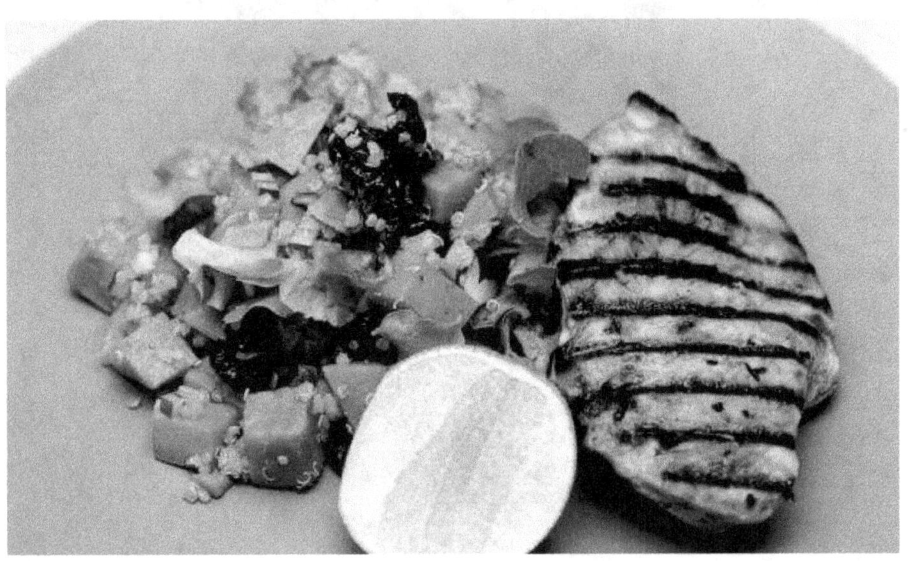

INGREDIENTS

-1 cup cooked quinoa
-1/2 grilled chicken breast
-1 cup mixed greens
-1/2 cup chopped cucumber
-1/4 cup chopped bell peppers
-balsamic vinaigrette dressing.

INSTRUCTIONS

1. Cook quinoa according to package directions.
2. Grill chicken breast and slice.
3. Combine quinoa, chicken, greens, cucumber, and bell peppers
4. Drizzle with vinaigrette.

NUTRITION INFO:

25% fat, 30% protein, 45% carbs, 500 calories.

Dinner: Baked Salmon with Roasted Vegetables

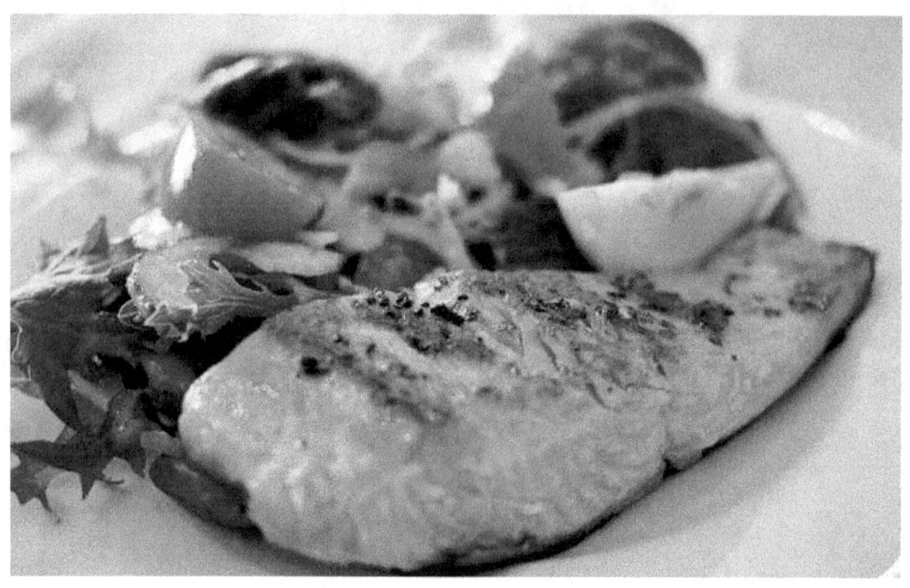

INGREDIENTS

-4 oz salmon filet

-1 tablespoon olive oil

-1 cup Brussels sprouts

-1/2 cup broccoli florets.

INSTRUCTIONS

1. Preheat the oven to 400°F.
2. Season salmon with salt and pepper.
3. Drizzle vegetables with olive oil and season.
4. Place salmon and vegetables on a baking sheet and roast for 15-20 minutes, or until salmon is cooked through.

NUTRITION INFO:

30% fat, 40% protein, 30% carbs, 450 calories.

Day 4
Breakfast: Tofu scrambled with onions and bell peppers

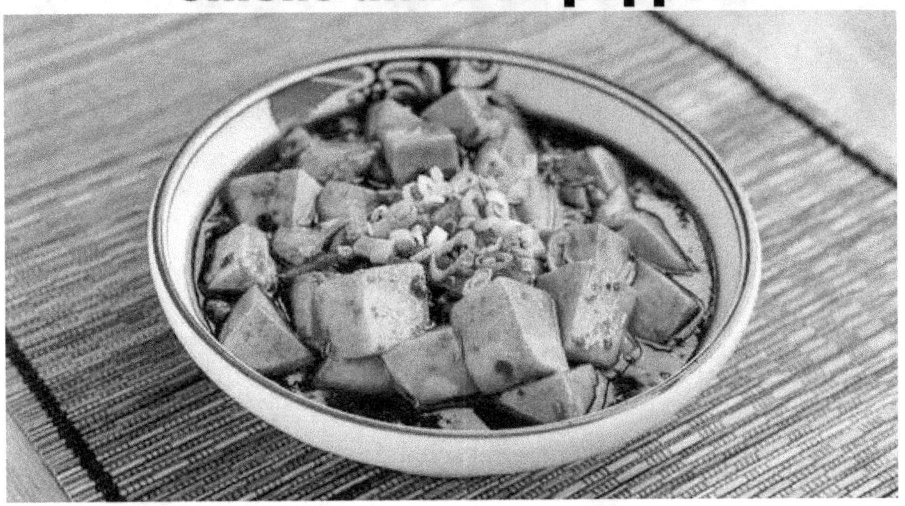

INGREDIENTS

-14 oz extra-firm tofu

-drained and pressed

-1 tablespoon olive oil

-1/2 medium onion, diced

-1 medium bell pepper

-diced (any color)

-1/4 cup chopped fresh herbs

(cilantro, parsley, or chives)

-1/4 teaspoon turmeric

-1/4 teaspoon smoked paprika

-Salt and pepper to taste

INSTRUCTIONS

1. Crumble the tofu into a bowl using your fingers or a fork.

2. Place olive oil in a big skillet and heat it over medium heat.

3. Cook for approximately five minutes, or until the onion is soft.

4. Add the bell pepper and cook until tender-crisp, about 5 more minutes. Stir in the turmeric, paprika, salt, and

and pepper.

5. Add the crumbled tofu and cook, stirring frequently, until heated through, about 5 minutes.

6. Before serving, mix in the fresh herbs.

NUTRITION INFO:

Calories: 350, Fat: 15g, Protein: 25g, Carbohydrates: 20g, Fiber: 5g

Lunch: Tuna salad lettuce wraps

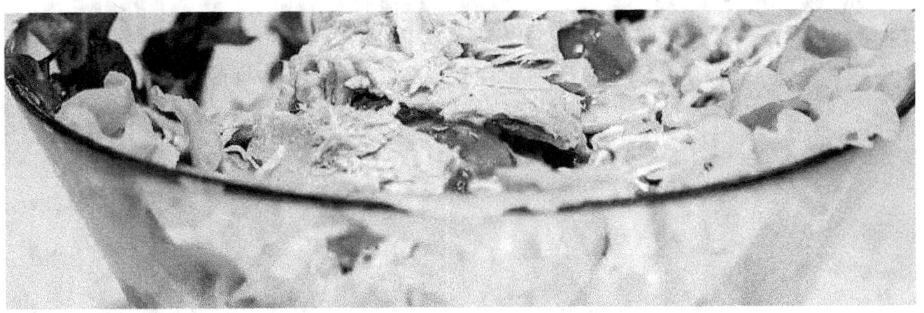

INGREDIENTS

-2 cans (5 oz each) of drained tuna in water.

-1/4 cup mayonnaise (Greek yogurt or avocado mayo for a lower-glycemic option).

-2 celery stalks, finely chopped.

-1/4 cup red onion, finely chopped. 2 tablespoons lemon juice.

-1 tablespoon chopped fresh herbs (dill, parsley, or chives).

-1/2 teaspoon Dijon mustard.

-Salt and pepper to taste. 8 large lettuce leaves (romaine, butter lettuce, or Boston bibb).

INSTRUCTIONS

1. In a large bowl, combine tuna, mayonnaise, celery, red onion, lemon juice, herbs, Dijon mustard, salt, and pepper.

2. Stir until well combined.

3. Wash and pat dry the lettuce leaves.

4. Spoon about 1/4 cup of tuna salad into the center of each lettuce leaf.

NUTRITION INFO:

Calories, 250 (using Greek yogurt mayo), Fat: 10g, Protein: 25g, Carbohydrates: 10g, Fiber: 2g

Dinner: Turkey meatballs with roasted sweet potato and Brussels sprouts

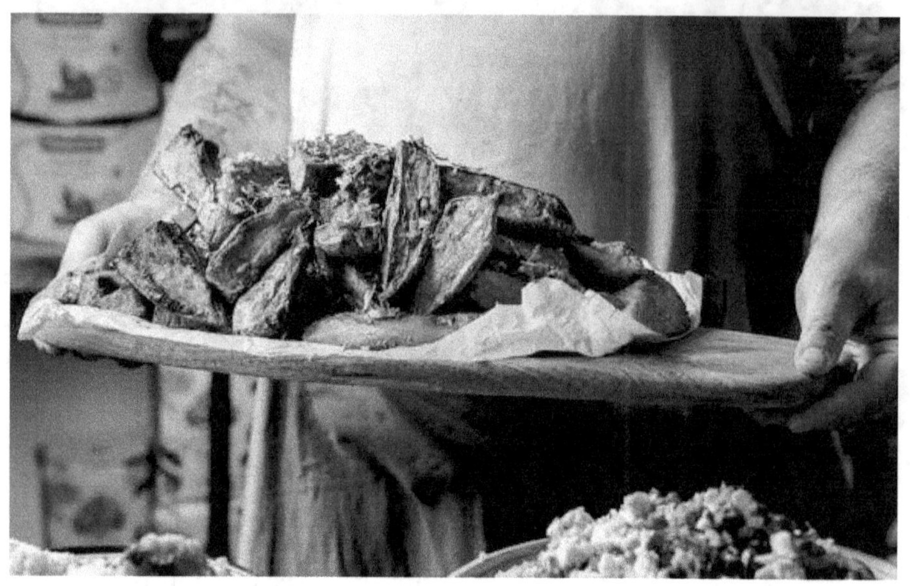

INGREDIENTS

Meatballs:
-1 lb ground turkey.
-1/2 cup rolled oats (quick or old-fashioned). -1/4 cup chopped fresh herbs (parsley, sage, or thyme).
-1/2 onion, finely chopped.
-1 egg.
-1/4 cup Dijon mustard.
-1 teaspoon garlic powder.
-1/2 teaspoon salt.
-1/4 teaspoon black pepper.

INSTRUCTIONS

1. Preheat the oven to 400°F (200°C).
2. A baking sheet should have parchment paper on one side.

Meatballs:
3. In a large bowl, combine ground turkey, oats, herbs, onion, egg, Dijon mustard, garlic powder, salt, and pepper.
4. Mix well until evenly incorporated and form into 12 meatballs.

-2 large sweet potatoes,
peeled and cubed.
-1 lb Brussels sprouts,
trimmed and halved.
-2 tablespoons of olive oil.
-1/2 teaspoon dried thyme.
-1/4 teaspoon salt.
-1/4 teaspoon black
pepper.

Vegetables:
6. Toss sweet potatoes and
Brussels sprouts with olive oil,
thyme, salt, and pepper.
7. Spread on the prepared
baking sheet.

Assemble: Arrange meatballs
evenly between the vegetables.
Roast: Bake for 25-30 minutes,
or until meatballs are cooked
through and vegetables are
tender and slightly browned.

NUTRITION INFO:

Calories: 450, Fat: 15g, Protein: 40g,
Carbohydrates: 50g, Fiber: 8g

Day 5
Breakfast: Almond milk, berries, and chia pudding

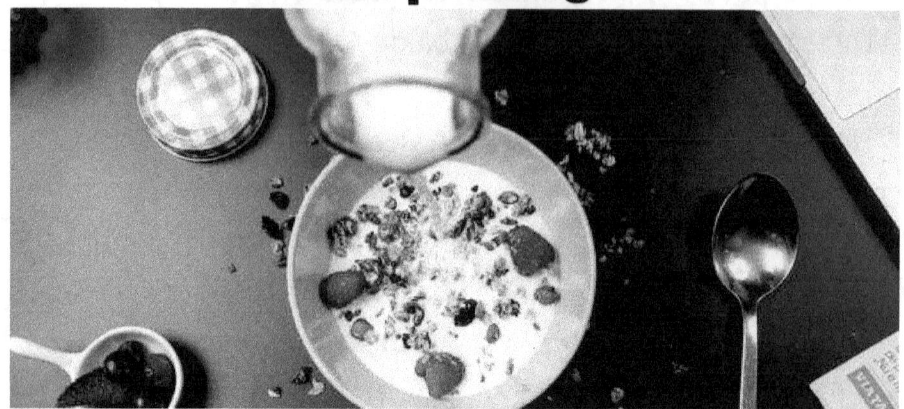

INGREDIENTS

-1/4 cup chia seeds.
-1 cup unsweetened almond milk.
1/2 tablespoon maple syrup or honey (optional).
-1/4 teaspoon vanilla extract (optional).
-1/2 cup of berries in various combinations (strawberries, blueberries, raspberries).

INSTRUCTIONS

1. In a small bowl or jar, whisk together chia seeds, almond milk, maple syrup or honey (if using), and vanilla extract (if using).
2. Give the mixture five minutes to settle so the chia seeds can absorb the liquid and become thicker.
3. Cover the bowl or jar and refrigerate for at least 4 hours, or overnight, for best results.
4. When ready to serve, stir in the berries.
5. You can enjoy the pudding as is or top it with additional toppings

like chopped nuts, shredded
coconut, or a drizzle of nut
butter.

NUTRITION INFO:

Calories: 250, Fat: 5g, Protein: 5g, Carbohydrates: 35g,
Fiber: 10g

Lunch: Lentil Soup & Whole-Wheat Bread

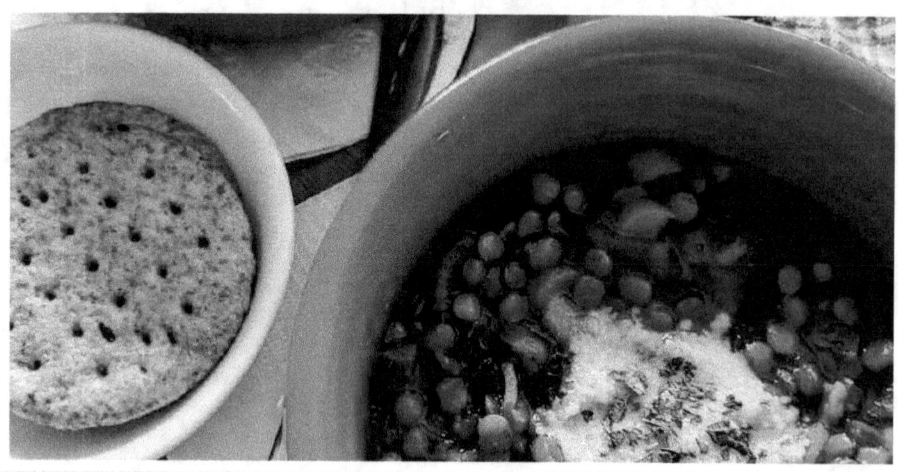

INGREDIENTS

- Olive oil.
- Onion, chopped.
- Carrots & celery, chopped.
- Garlic, minced.
- Green lentils, rinsed.
- Vegetable broth.
- Diced tomatoes, undrained.
- Dried thyme & oregano.
- Salt & pepper.
- Whole-wheat bread.
- Olive oil (optional).

INSTRUCTIONS

1. Sauté onion, carrots, & celery in olive oil until softened.
2. Add garlic, lentils, broth, tomatoes, herbs, & seasonings.
3. Lentils should be simmered for 30 minutes or until soft.
4. Toast whole-wheat bread (optional) and drizzle with olive oil (optional).

NUTRITION INFO:

Calories: 300, Fat: 5g, Protein: 15g, Carbohydrates: 40g, Fiber: 5g

Dinner: Shrimp scampi with zucchini noodles

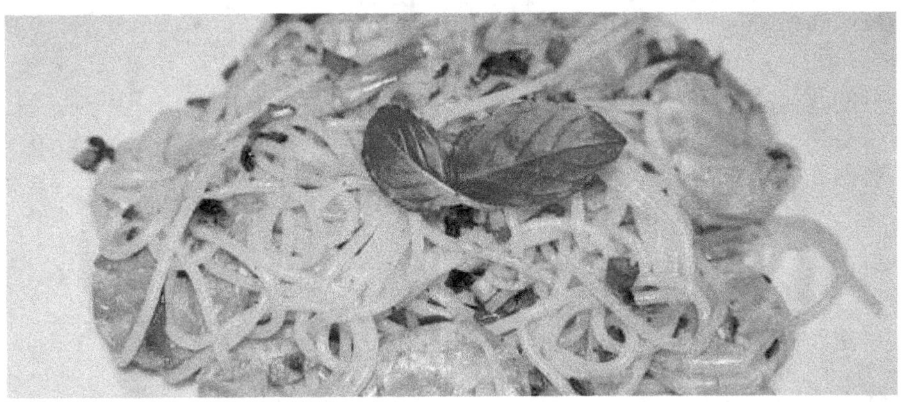

INGREDIENTS

-1 lb large shrimp, peeled and deveined.
-1 tablespoon olive oil
-2 cloves garlic, minced
-1/4 cup dry white wine (optional)
-1/2 cup chicken or vegetable broth
-1/4 cup chopped fresh parsley
-1/4 teaspoon red pepper flakes (optional)
-Salt and pepper to taste
-2 large zucchini, spiralized into noodles

INSTRUCTIONS

1. Spread the olive oil in a big skillet and place it over medium heat. Sauté the garlic for 30 seconds or until it begins to smell aromatic.

2. Add the shrimp and cook until they turn pink and opaque, about 2-3 minutes per side.

3. Deglaze the pan with white wine (if using) by scraping up any browned bits with a spatula. Let the wine simmer for a minute until slightly reduced.

4. After adding the chicken or

vegetable broth, boil the
mixture.
5. Stir in parsley, red pepper
flakes (if using), salt, and
pepper.
6. Add the zucchini noodles
and cook for just 1-2 minutes,
until slightly softened but still
al dente.

NUTRITION INFO:

Calories: 350, Fat: 15g, Protein: 30g, Carbohydrates: 20g,
Fiber: 3g

Day 6
Breakfast: Greek yogurt with rolled oats and cinnamon

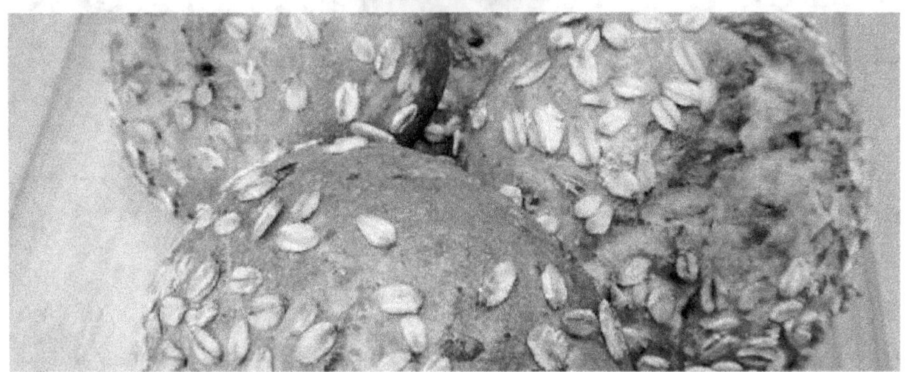

INGREDIENTS

-1 cup plain Greek yogurt (choose low-fat or full-fat, depending on your preference)
-1/4 cup rolled oats (quick or old-fashioned)
-1/2 teaspoon ground cinnamon
-Optional toppings: fresh berries, chopped nuts, chia seeds, honey (use sparingly)

INSTRUCTIONS

1. In a bowl, combine Greek yogurt, rolled oats, and cinnamon.
2. Stir well and let sit for 5-10 minutes, allowing the oats to soften and absorb the yogurt's liquid. This creates a creamier texture.
3. Top with your favorite low-glycemic options like fresh berries (blueberries, raspberries, strawberries), chopped nuts (almonds, walnuts, pecans), chia seeds, or a drizzle of honey if desired.

NUTRITION INFO:

Calories: 250, Fat: 5g, Protein: 20g Carbohydrates: 25g, Fiber: 5g

Lunch: Chicken stir-fry with brown rice and vegetables

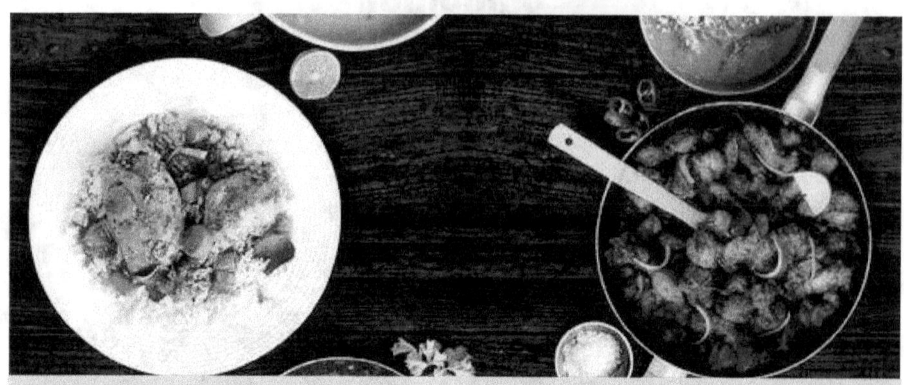

INGREDIENTS

-1 lb boneless, skinless chicken breasts, sliced
-1 tablespoon olive oil
-1 bag frozen mixed vegetables (broccoli, carrots, bell peppers)
-1/2 cup low-sodium chicken broth
-2 tablespoons soy sauce (reduced sodium)
-1 tablespoon rice vinegar
-1/2 teaspoon black pepper
-1 cup cooked brown rice

INSTRUCTIONS

1. The olive oil should be heated over medium-high heat in a large skillet or wok.
2. Add chicken and cook until browned and cooked through, about 5 minutes.
3. Add frozen vegetables and cook until thawed and slightly tender, about 5 minutes.
4. Pour in broth, soy sauce, rice vinegar, and black pepper. After bringing to a simmer, cook for one minute.

NUTRITION INFO:

Calories: 450, Fat: 15g, Protein: 40g, Carbohydrates: 45g, Fiber: 8g

Dinner: Veggie chili with quinoa

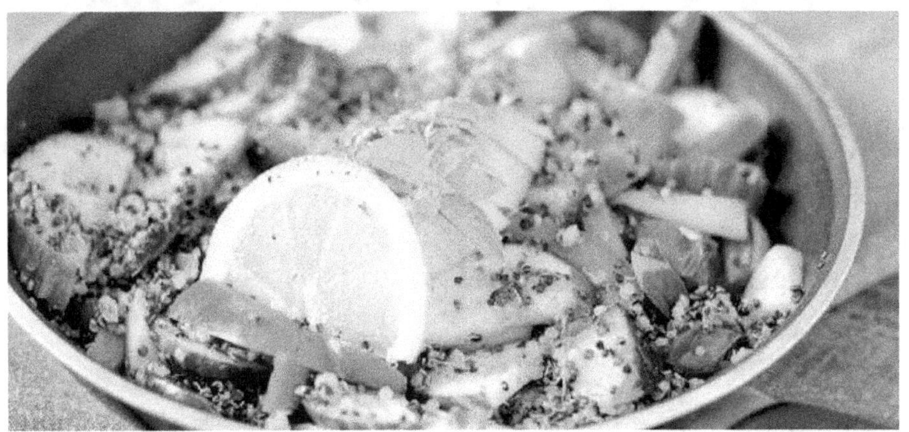

INGREDIENTS

-1 tablespoon olive oil

-1 onion, chopped

-2 cloves garlic, minced

-1 bell pepper, chopped (any color)

-2 carrots, chopped

-2 celery stalks, chopped

-1 (15 oz) can diced tomatoes, undrained

-1 (14.5 ounce can of washed and drained black beans

-1 can (14.5 oz) of rinsed and drained kidney beans

-1 (14.5 oz) can corn, drained (optional)

-4 cups vegetable broth

INSTRUCTIONS

1. In a big pot or Dutch oven, warm up the olive oil over medium heat. Add the onion and simmer for about 5 minutes, or until softened.

2. Add garlic, bell pepper, carrots, and celery. 3. Cook for 5 more minutes, or until vegetables are slightly softened.

4. Stir in diced tomatoes, black beans, kidney beans, corn (if using), vegetable broth, chili powder, cumin, smoked paprika, salt, and pepper.

5. Bring to a boil, then reduce heat to low and simmer for 30 minutes, or until flavors are melded.

-1 cup cooked quinoa
-1 teaspoon chili powder
-1/2 teaspoon cumin
-1/4 teaspoon smoked
paprika
-Salt and pepper to taste

Toppings (optional):
chopped avocado,
chopped cilantro, low-fat
sour cream, hot sauce, lime
wedges

NUTRITION INFO:

Calories: 450, Fat: 15g,
Protein: 40g,
Carbohydrates: 45g, Fiber:
8g

Day 7
Breakfast: Whole-wheat toast with avocado and hemp seeds

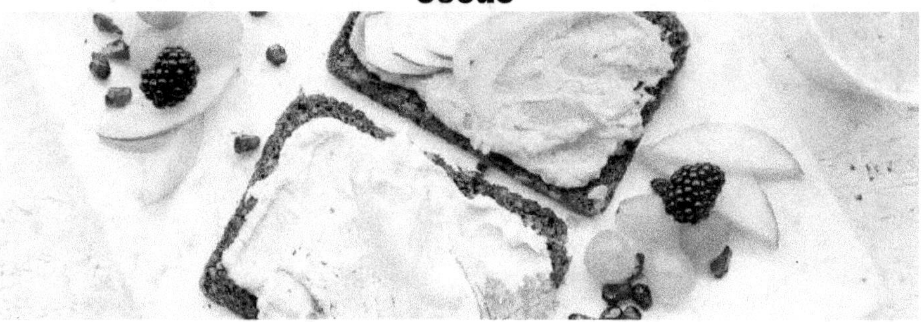

INGREDIENTS

-2 slices whole-wheat bread

-1/2 ripe avocado

-1 tablespoon hemp seeds

-Squeeze of lemon juice (optional)

-Salt and pepper to taste

Optional additions:

-Sliced tomato

-Chopped red onion

-Chili flakes

-Hot sauce

-Fresh herbs like cilantro or parsley

INSTRUCTIONS

1. Toast the whole-wheat bread to your desired level of crispness.
2. While the bread is toasting, mash the avocado in a bowl with a fork to your preferred consistency.
3. Top the toast with a layer of mashed avocado.
4. Sprinkle the hemp seeds over the avocado.
If preferred, squeeze in some lemon juice.
5. To taste, add salt and pepper for seasoning.

NUTRITION INFO:

Calories: 250, Fat: 15g

Protein: 8g, Carbohydrates: 25g, Fiber: 5g

Lunch: Black Bean Burgers on whole-wheat Buns

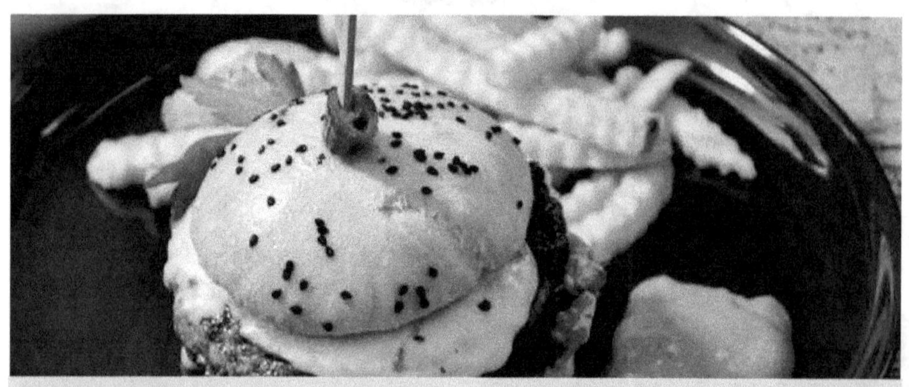

INGREDIENTS

For the Burgers

-A 15-oz can of black beans that have been cleaned and emptied
-1/2 cup rolled oats (quick or old-fashioned)
-1/4 cup chopped onion
-1/4 cup chopped red bell pepper
-2 cloves garlic, minced
-1 egg
-1/4 cup chopped cilantro
-1 tablespoon olive oil
-1 teaspoon chili powder
-1/2 teaspoon cumin

INSTRUCTIONS

1. Preheat the oven to 400°F (200°C). Put parchment paper on a baking pan.
2. In a large bowl, mash the black beans with a fork until slightly chunky.
3. Add oats, onion, bell pepper, garlic, egg, cilantro, olive oil, chili powder, cumin, paprika, salt, and pepper. Mix well until combined.
5. Form the mixture into 4 equal patties.
6. Put the patties onto the baking sheet that has been ready.
7. Bake for 20 to 25 minutes, or until well cooked and golden brown.

-1/4 teaspoon smoked paprika
-Salt and pepper to taste

For the Buns:

-2 whole-wheat hamburger buns
-Optional toppings: lettuce, tomato, avocado, onion, salsa, vegan mayo

8. Toast the whole-wheat buns.

NUTRITION INFO:

Calories: 400, Fat: 15g, Protein: 25g, Carbohydrates: 40g, Fiber: 8g

Dinner: Salmon with roasted asparagus and quinoa

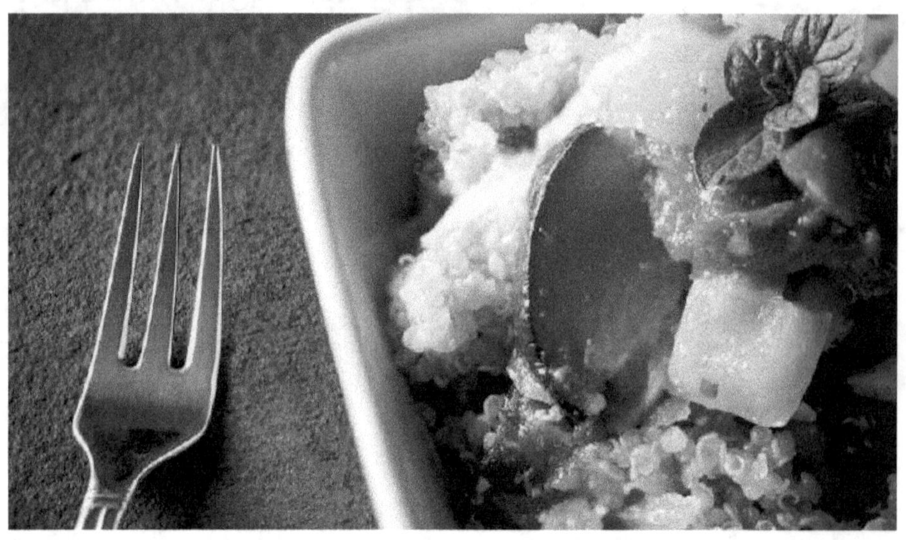

INGREDIENTS

-2 salmon filets (6 oz each)

-1 tbsp olive oil

-1/2 tsp each salt and pepper

-1 bunch asparagus, trimmed and halved

-1/4 cup quinoa, rinsed

-1 cup vegetable broth

-1/2 lemon, sliced (optional)

INSTRUCTIONS

1. Preheat the oven to 400°F (200°C). Put parchment paper on a baking pan.

2. Season salmon with olive oil, salt, and pepper.

3. Toss asparagus with olive oil, salt, and pepper. Spread on the prepared baking sheet.

4. Roast asparagus for 10-12 minutes, or until tender-crisp.

5. While asparagus roasts, cook quinoa according to package instructions.

Usually, it's 1:2 quinoa to water ratio, brought to a boil, then simmered for 15 minutes. 6. In the last 5 minutes of quinoa cooking, add the salmon filets nestled in the quinoa. Cover and steam until salmon is cooked through and flakes easily (about 12-15 minutes).

NUTRITION INFO:

Calories: 450, Fat: 20g, Protein: 35g, Carbohydrates: 40g, Fiber: 5g

1. kale, feta, and egg burrito

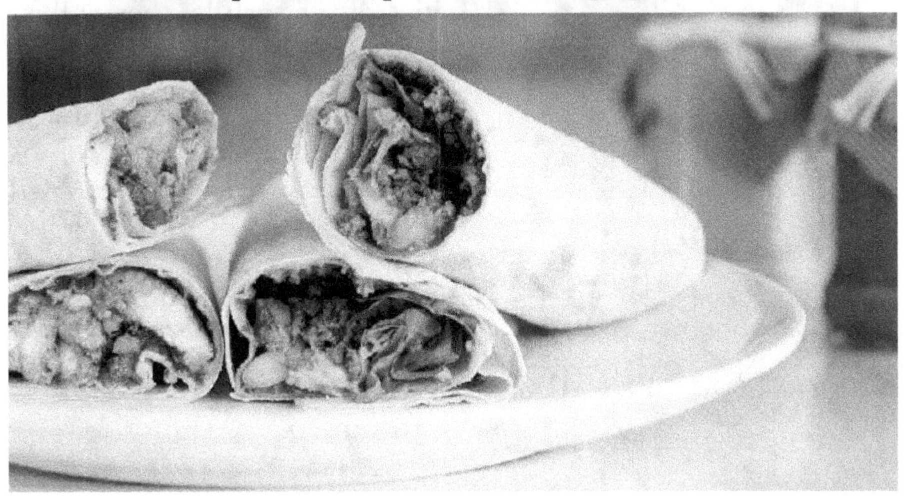

INGREDIENTS

- 2 large kale leaves, cut after the stems are removed
- 2 eggs
- 1/4 cup crumbled feta cheese
- 2 whole-grain or low-carb tortillas
- 1 tablespoon olive oil
- Salt and pepper to taste

INSTRUCTIONS

1. Prepare the Kale: Heat olive oil in a pan over medium heat. Add chopped kale and sauté for 2-3 minutes until wilted. Season with a pinch of salt and pepper. Set aside.

2. Scramble the Eggs: In the same pan, scramble the eggs until fully cooked. Add pepper and salt according to taste.

3. Assemble the Burrito: Warm the tortillas in the microwave or on a skillet for a few seconds. Place the cooked kale on each tortilla,

followed by the scrambled eggs. Sprinkle crumbled feta cheese evenly on top.

4. Roll the Burrito: Fold in the sides of the tortilla, then roll it up tightly to enclose the filling.

5. Serve: Cut the burrito in half diagonally and serve warm.

NUTRITION INFO:

Calories: 300-350, Carbohydrates: 20-25g, Fiber: 5-8g, Protein: 15-20g, Fat: 15-20g

2. mashed sweet potato breakfast bowl

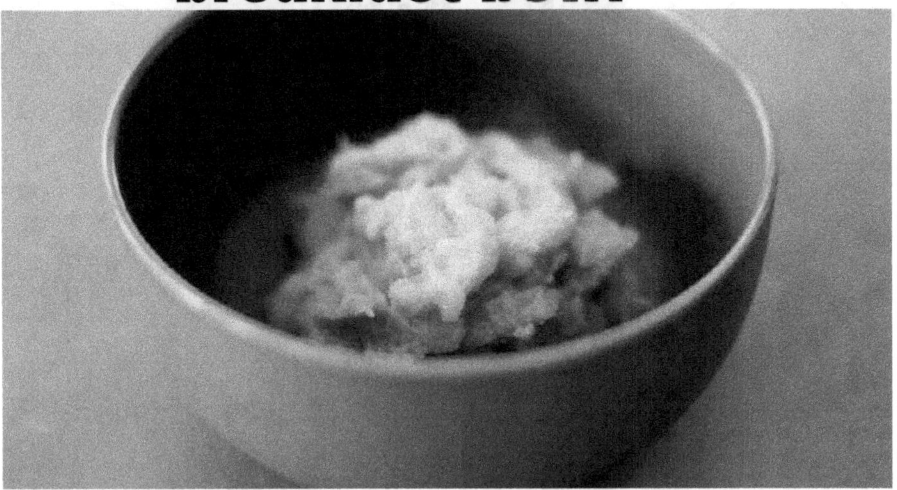

INGREDIENTS

- 1 medium-sized sweet potato
- 2 eggs
- 1/2 avocado, sliced
- 1/4 cup diced tomatoes
- 2 tablespoons chopped fresh cilantro
- Salt and pepper to taste
- For frying, use cooking spray or olive oil.

INSTRUCTIONS

1. Prepare the Sweet Potato: Pierce the sweet potato a few times with a fork. Microwave it for 4-6 minutes or until it's tender all the way through. Alternatively, you can bake it in the oven at 400°F (200°C) for about 45-60 minutes.

2. Smash the Sweet Potato: Once the sweet potato is cooked, slice it open and scoop the flesh into a bowl. Use a fork to mash it lightly.

3. Cook the Eggs: Heat a pan over medium heat and add a bit of olive oil or cooking spray.

4. Crack the eggs into the pan and cook them to your desired doneness (fried, scrambled, or poached). Season with salt and pepper.

5. Assemble the Bowl: Divide the smashed sweet potato into two bowls. Top each bowl with a cooked egg, sliced avocado, diced tomatoes, and chopped cilantro.

6. Season and Serve: Season with additional salt and pepper if desired. Enjoy your nutritious and flavorful smashed sweet potato breakfast bowl!

NUTRITION INFO:

3. chickpea omelet with asparagus

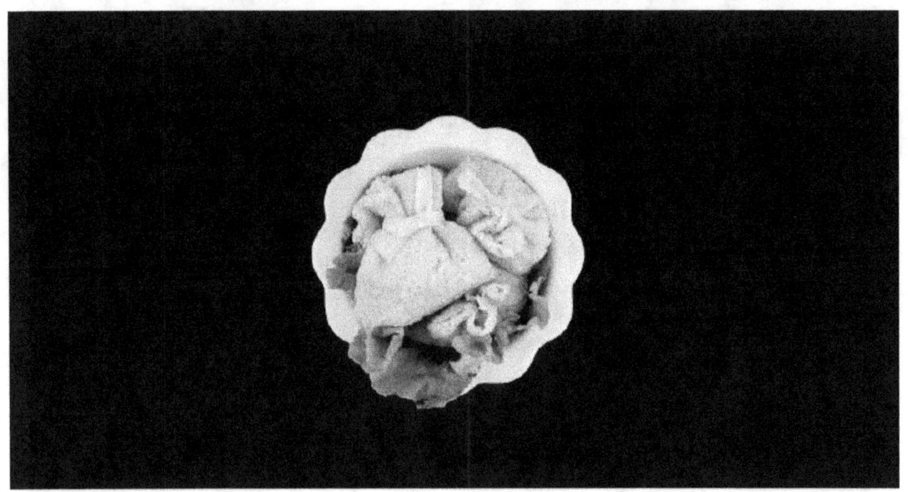

INGREDIENTS

- 1/2 cup chickpea flour
- 1/2 cup water
- 1/4 teaspoon baking powder
- Salt and pepper to taste
- 1/2 cup chopped asparagus
- 1/4 cup diced onion
- 1 tablespoon olive oil
- Optional: 2 tablespoons nutritional yeast for a cheesy flavor

INSTRUCTIONS

1. Prepare the Chickpea Batter: In a mixing bowl, combine chickpea flour, water, baking powder, salt, and pepper. Whisk until a smooth batter forms. If using nutritional yeast, add it to the batter for a cheesy taste.

2. Sauté the Asparagus and Onion: Heat olive oil in a pan over medium heat. Add chopped asparagus and diced onion. Sauté for about 3-4 minutes until they're slightly tender. Season with salt and pepper.

Chickpea flour is a great alternative to eggs for those looking for a plant-based option. It's high in protein and fiber, which can help in managing glycemic load. Adjust seasoning and ingredients according to your taste preferences.

3. Cook the Chickpea Omelette: Pour half of the chickpea batter into the pan, swirling it around to spread evenly. Cook for 2-3 minutes until the edges start to set.

4. Add Asparagus and Onion: Sprinkle half of the sautéed asparagus and onion mixture on one side of the omelet.

5. Fold and Serve: Gently fold the other half of the omelet over the filling. Cook for an additional minute or until the omelet is fully set.

6. Repeat for the Second Omelet: Repeat the process with the remaining batter and asparagus mixture to make the second omelet.

7. Serve: Slide the omelets onto plates and garnish with fresh herbs if desired. Enjoy your chickpea omelets with asparagus.

4. cinnamon pear oatmeal bowl

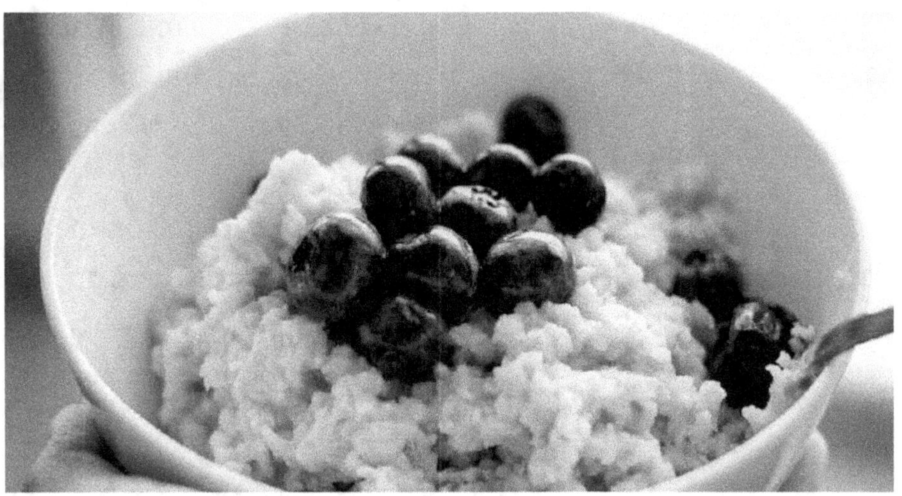

INGREDIENTS

- 1/2 cup rolled oats (old-fashioned oats)
- 1 cup unsweetened almond milk (or any preferred milk)
- 1 medium ripe pear, diced
- 1/2 teaspoon ground cinnamon
- 1 tablespoon chopped walnuts (optional)
- 1 teaspoon of optionally sweetened maple syrup or honey

INSTRUCTIONS

1. Cook the Oats: In a small saucepan, combine the rolled oats and almond milk. Turn the heat down to low after bringing to a gentle boil over medium heat. Simmer for about 5-7 minutes, stirring occasionally, until the oats are cooked and creamy.

2. Add Pear and Cinnamon: Stir in the diced pear and ground cinnamon into the cooked oatmeal. Cook for an additional 2-3 minutes until the pear softens slightly and the flavors meld together.

3. Sweeten (if desired): If you prefer additional sweetness, drizzle honey or maple syrup over the oatmeal and mix well. Adjust sweetness according to your taste.

4. Serve: Transfer the oatmeal to a bowl. Top it with chopped walnuts for added crunch and nutrients.

NUTRITION INFO:

Calories: 300-350, Carbohydrates: 50-60g, Fiber: 8-10g, Protein: 5-7g, Fat: 8-10g

5. black bean egg white omelet

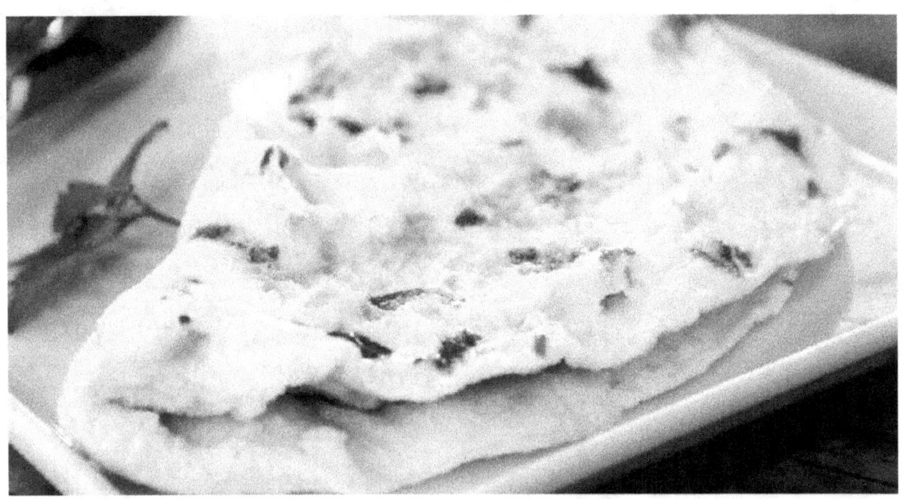

INGREDIENTS

- Half a cup of black beans, washed and drained
- 3 egg whites
- 1/4 cup diced tomatoes
- 1/4 cup of bell peppers, chopped, any color
- 1 tablespoon chopped cilantro
- 1 tablespoon olive oil
- Salt and pepper to taste
- Optional: 2 tablespoons shredded low-fat cheese

INSTRUCTIONS

1. Prepare the Black Beans: In a small bowl, lightly mash the black beans with a fork. Set aside.
2. Whisk the Egg Whites: In another bowl, whisk the egg whites until frothy. Season with a pinch of salt and pepper.
3. Sauté the Vegetables: Heat olive oil in a non-stick skillet over medium heat. Add diced tomatoes and bell peppers, sautéing for 2-3 minutes until they soften.
4. Add Egg Whites and Beans: Pour the whisked egg whites into the skillet, swirling to

cover the vegetables evenly. Allow the eggs to set slightly.

5. Sprinkle Beans and Cilantro: Spread the mashed black beans evenly over half of the omelet. Sprinkle chopped cilantro on top. Optionally, add shredded low-fat cheese.

6. Fold and Cook: Gently fold the other half of the omelet over the filling. Cook for an additional minute or until the omelet is fully set.

7. Serve: Slide the omelet onto a plate and garnish with extra cilantro if desired.

NUTRITION INFO:

Calories: 200-250, Carbohydrates: 20-25g, Fiber: 6-8g, Protein: 15-18g, Fat: 6-8g

Lunch and dinner
1. cucumber and pepper tabbouleh with chicken

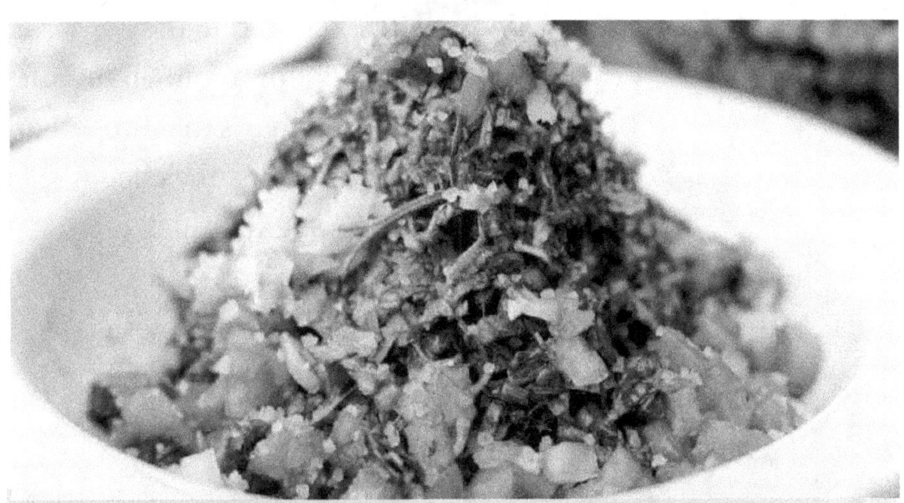

INGREDIENTS

- 1 cup cooked quinoa (cooled)
- 1 cup diced cucumber
- 1 cup of chopped bell peppers, any color
- 1 cup chopped cooked chicken breast
- 1/4 cup chopped fresh parsley
- 1/4 cup chopped fresh mint leaves
- 2 tablespoons olive oil
- 2 tablespoons lemon juice
- Salt and pepper to taste

INSTRUCTIONS

1. Prepare the Ingredients: In a large mixing bowl, combine the cooked quinoa, diced cucumber, diced bell peppers, chopped cooked chicken breast, chopped parsley, and chopped mint leaves.

2. Make the Dressing: In a small bowl, whisk together the olive oil and lemon juice. Tailor the salt and pepper to your personal preference.

3. Combine Ingredients: Pour the

dressing over the quinoa mixture. Gently toss until the dressing coats all of the ingredients.

4. Chill (Optional): If time allows, refrigerate the tabbouleh for about 30 minutes to let the flavors meld together.

5. Serve: Divide the cucumber and pepper tabbouleh into serving bowls or plates. Optionally, garnish with additional parsley or mint leaves for presentation.

NUTRITION INFO:

Calories: 300-35p0, Carbohydrates: 20-25g, Fiber: 3-5g, Protein: 20-25g, Fat: 15-18g

2. chicken and cilantro lime quinoa bowl

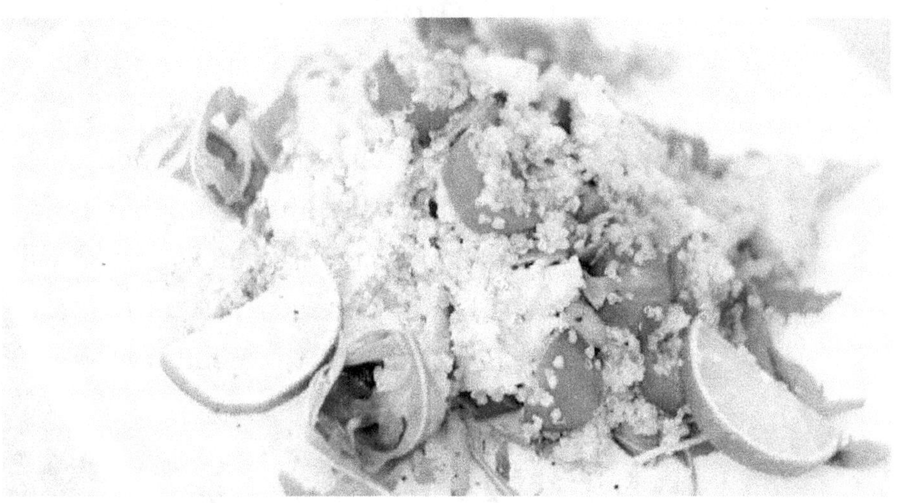

INGREDIENTS

- 1 cup cooked quinoa (cooled)
- 8 oz (about 225g) cooked chicken breast, diced or shredded
- 1 cup diced cherry tomatoes
- 1/2 cup diced red onion
- 1/4 cup chopped fresh cilantro
- Lime juice (1-2) (tailor to taste)
- 2 tablespoons olive oil
- Salt and pepper to taste

INSTRUCTIONS

1. Prepare the Ingredients: In a mixing bowl, combine the cooked quinoa, diced chicken breast, diced cherry tomatoes, diced red onion, and chopped cilantro.

2. Make the Dressing: In a small bowl, whisk together the lime juice and olive oil. Tailor the salt and pepper to your personal preference.

3. Combine Ingredients: Pour the dressing over the quinoa and chicken mixture. Gently toss until the dressing coats all of the ingredients.

4. Chill (Optional): If time allows, refrigerate the quinoa bowl for about 15-30 minutes to allow the flavors to meld together.

5. Serve: Divide the chicken and cilantro lime quinoa mixture into serving bowls or plates. Optionally, garnish with additional cilantro or lime wedges for presentation.

NUTRITION INFO:

Calories: 350-400, Carbohydrates: 25-30g, Fiber: 3-5g, Protein: 25-30g, Fat: 15-20g

3. chicken, kale, and avocado bowl

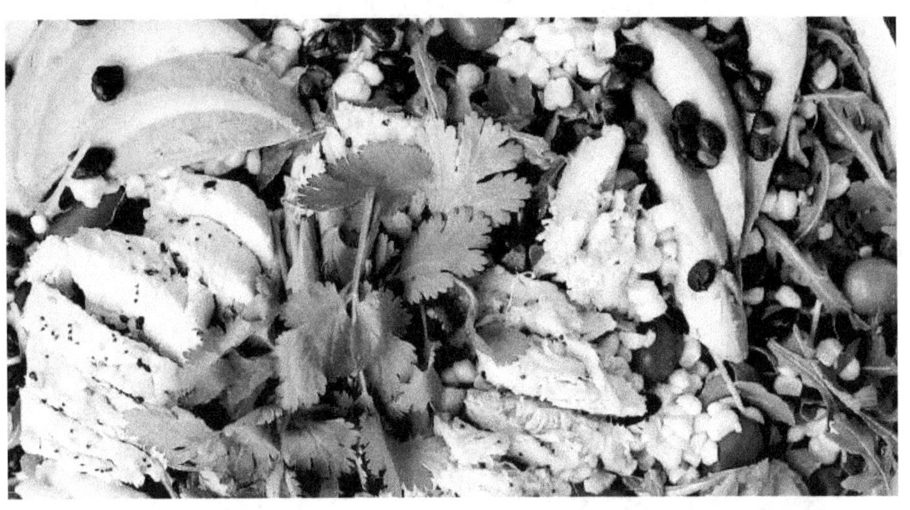

INGREDIENTS

- 8 oz (about 225g) cooked chicken breast, sliced or diced
- 2 cups of finely chopped, stem-free kale leaves
- 1 ripe avocado, sliced
- 1/4 cup diced red onion
- 2 tablespoons olive oil
- 2 tablespoons lemon juice
- Salt and pepper to taste
- Optional: 2 tablespoons chopped nuts (such as almonds or walnuts)

INSTRUCTIONS

1. Prepare the Ingredients: In a mixing bowl, combine the chopped kale, diced red onion, and sliced avocado.

2. Make the Dressing: In a small bowl, whisk together the olive oil and lemon juice. Tailor the salt and pepper to your personal preference.

3. Massage the Kale: Pour the dressing over the kale and massage it gently with your hands for a minute or two. The kale leaves get softer as a result.

4. Assemble the Bowl: Divide the dressed kale mixture into serving bowls. Top each bowl with the cooked chicken breast slices or cubes.

5. Garnish and Serve: Optionally, sprinkle chopped nuts over the bowls for added texture and nutrients.

NUTRITION INFO:

Calories: 350-400, Carbohydrates: 10-15g, Fiber: 6-8g, Protein: 25-30g, Fat: 20-25g

4. tuna, spinach, and feta pita wrap

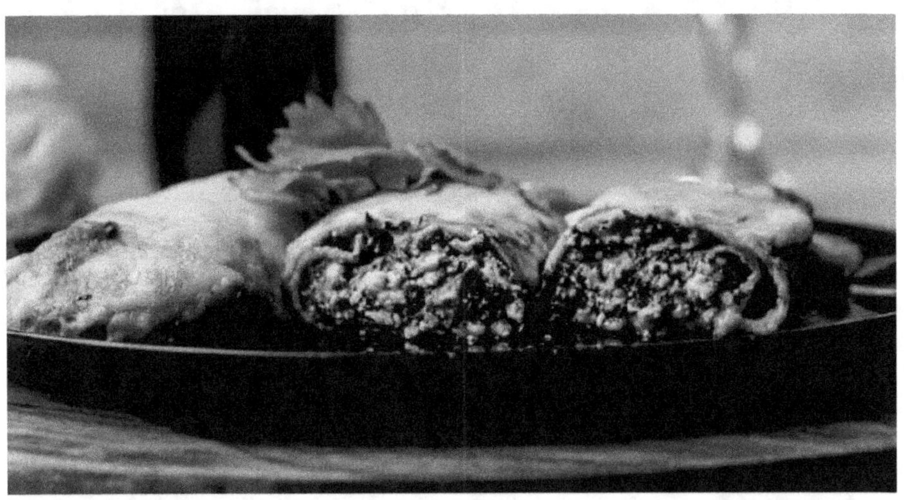

INGREDIENTS

- 1 whole-grain pita pocket (or low-carb pita for a lower glycemic option)
- 1 drained 5-ounce can of tuna
- 1 cup fresh spinach leaves
- 2 tablespoons crumbled feta cheese
- 1 tablespoon olive oil
- 1 tablespoon lemon juice
- Salt and pepper to taste

INSTRUCTIONS

1. Prepare the Ingredients: If using a whole-grain pita pocket, slightly warm it to make it more pliable.

2. Make the Tuna Mixture: In a mixing bowl, combine the drained tuna, fresh spinach leaves, crumbled feta cheese, olive oil, lemon juice, salt, and pepper. Mix until well combined.

3. Assemble the Wrap: Lay the warm pita flat and spoon the tuna mixture onto the center of the pita.

4. Fold and Roll: Fold the sides of the pita

over the filling, then roll it up tightly like a wrap.

5. Slice and Serve: Slice the wrap in half diagonally and serve.

NUTRITION INFO:

Calories: 300-350, Carbohydrates: 20-25g, Fiber: 5-8g, Protein: 20-25g, Fat: 15-20g

5. sushi bowl

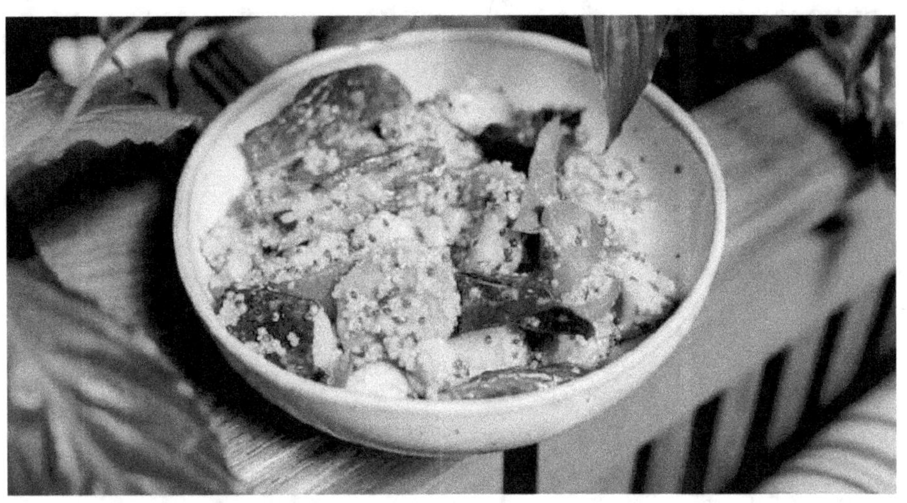

INGREDIENTS

- 1 cup cooked quinoa or cauliflower rice (for a lower carb option)
- 4 oz (about 113g) raw sushi-grade salmon or tuna, thinly sliced
- 1/2 avocado, sliced
- 1/2 cucumber, thinly sliced
- 1 small carrot, julienned
- 1 tablespoon of white or black sesame seeds
- 2 tablespoons low-sodium soy sauce or tamari

INSTRUCTIONS

1. Prepare the Base: Divide the cooked quinoa or cauliflower rice between serving bowls as the base.

2. Assemble the Bowl: Arrange the sliced salmon or tuna, avocado, cucumber, and julienned carrot over the quinoa/cauliflower rice in separate sections, creating a visually appealing layout.

3. Make the Sauce: In a small bowl, mix the low-sodium soy sauce or tamari with rice vinegar and sesame oil (if using). Adjust the ratios to your taste preference.

4. Drizzle Sauce and Garnish:

- 1 tablespoon rice vinegar
- 1 teaspoon sesame oil
(optional)
- 1 green onion, thinly
sliced (for garnish)
- Nori seaweed strips
(optional)

Drizzle the sauce over the sushi bowl ingredients. Overtop, scatter chopped green onions and sesame seeds. Add nori seaweed strips for an extra sushi-like touch.

5. Serve: Serve immediately and enjoy your nutritious and flavorful sushi bowl

NUTRITION INFO:

Calories: 350-400, Carbohydrates: 20-25g, Fiber: 5-8g, Protein: 25-30g, Fat: 15-20g

6. chicken and cream cheese wrap

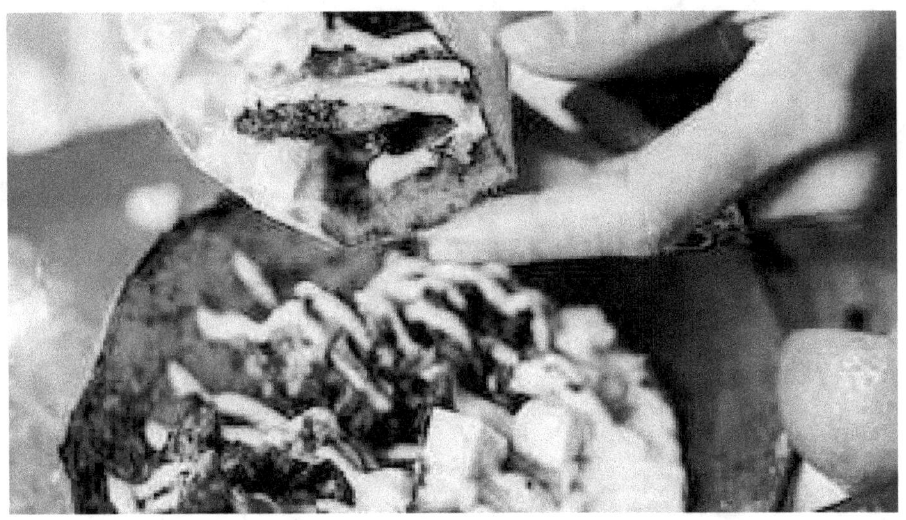

INGREDIENTS

- 1 whole-grain or low-carb wrap (choose one with lower glycemic impact)
- 4 oz (about 113g) cooked chicken breast, sliced or shredded
- 2 tablespoons low-fat cream cheese
- 1/4 cup sliced cucumbers
- 1/4 cup shredded lettuce or spinach
- Salt and pepper to taste

INSTRUCTIONS

1. Prepare the Wrap: Lay the whole-grain or low-carb wrap flat on a clean surface.

2. Spread Cream Cheese: Spread the low-fat cream cheese evenly over the surface of the wrap.

3. Layer Ingredients: Arrange the cooked chicken breast slices or shredded chicken on top of the cream cheese. Add sliced cucumbers and shredded lettuce or spinach.

4. Season and Roll: Season with salt and pepper to taste. Roll the wrap tightly, starting from one

end, enclosing the filling.

5. Slice and Serve: Slice the wrap in half diagonally and serve.

NUTRITION INFO:

Calories: 300-350, Carbohydrates: 20-25g, Fiber: 3-5g, Protein: 25-30g, Fat: 10-15g

7. cheeseburger salad

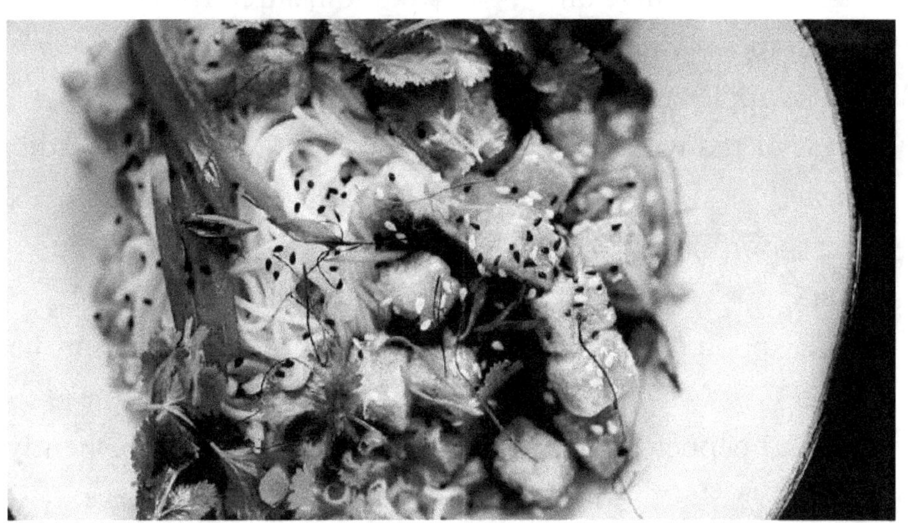

INGREDIENTS

- 8 oz (about 225g) lean ground beef or turkey
- 4 cups mixed salad greens (lettuce, spinach, etc.)
- 1/2 cup cherry tomatoes, halved
- 1/4 cup diced red onion
- 1/4 cup shredded cheddar cheese (choose low-fat if preferred)
- 2 tablespoons diced pickles
- 2 tablespoons chopped green onions (optional)
- Salt and pepper to taste

INSTRUCTIONS

1. Cook the Ground Beef or Turkey: In a skillet over medium heat, cook the lean ground beef or turkey until fully cooked. Season with salt and pepper to taste. Once cooked, set it aside to cool slightly.

2. Prepare the Dressing: In a small bowl, whisk together the olive oil, vinegar, Dijon mustard, garlic powder, salt, and pepper to create the salad dressing.

3. Assemble the Salad: In a large mixing bowl, combine the mixed salad greens,

Dressing Ingredients:
- 2 tablespoons olive oil
- 1 tablespoon vinegar (such as apple cider vinegar or red wine vinegar)
- 1 teaspoon Dijon mustard
- 1/2 teaspoon garlic powder
- Salt and pepper to taste

halved cherry tomatoes, diced red onion, shredded cheddar cheese, diced pickles, and chopped green onions.

4. Add the Cooked Meat: Add the slightly cooled cooked ground beef or turkey to the salad mixture.

5. Toss with Dressing: Pour the prepared dressing over the salad and meat mixture. Gently toss until everything is evenly coated with the dressing.

6. Serve: Divide the cheeseburger salad into serving bowls or plates.

NUTRITION INFO:

Calories: 300-350, Carbohydrates: 6-8g, Fiber: 2-3g, Protein: 25-30g, Fat: 20-25g

Snacks
1. Sunbutter pumpkin protein balls

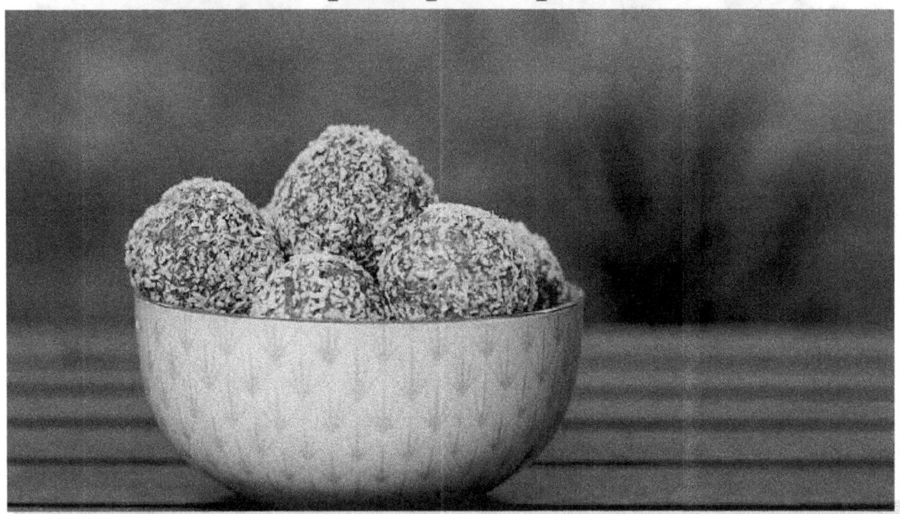

INGREDIENTS

- 1 cup pumpkin puree
- 1/2 cup sunflower seed butter (sunbutter)
- 1/4 cup unsweetened shredded coconut
- 1/4 cup protein powder (vanilla or unflavored)
- 2 tablespoons chia seeds
- 1 teaspoon ground cinnamon
- 1/4 teaspoon ground nutmeg
- 1/4 teaspoon ground ginger

INSTRUCTIONS

1. Mix Ingredients: In a mixing bowl, combine the pumpkin puree, sunflower seed butter, unsweetened shredded coconut, protein powder, chia seeds, ground cinnamon, ground nutmeg, and ground ginger. If you prefer extra sweetness, add honey or maple syrup to taste.

2. Combine Thoroughly: Mix all the ingredients together until a uniform dough forms. If the mixture is too wet, add more protein powder or shredded

- 1-2 tablespoons honey or maple syrup (optional for sweetness)
- Additional shredded coconut or chopped nuts for coating (optional)

coconut. If too dry, add a touch more pumpkin puree or sunflower seed butter.

3. Form Balls: Using your hands, roll the mixture into bite-sized balls, about 1 inch in diameter. If desired, roll each ball in additional shredded coconut or chopped nuts for coating.

4. Chill and Set: Place the protein balls on a baking sheet lined with parchment paper and refrigerate them for at least 30 minutes to set.

5. Serve or Store: Once set, these protein balls can be served immediately or stored in an airtight container in the refrigerator for up to a week.

NUTRITION INFO:

Calories: 120-150, Carbohydrates: 7-10g, Fiber: 3-5g, Protein: 5-7g, Fat: 8-10g

2. Taco-spiced chickpeas

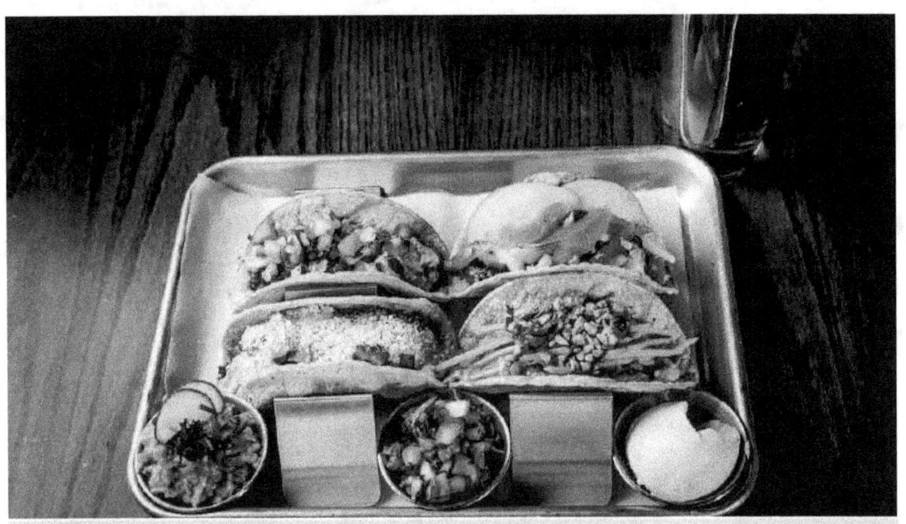

INGREDIENTS

- 2 cans (15 oz each) chickpeas, drained and rinsed
- 2 tablespoons olive oil
- 1 tablespoon chili powder
- 1 teaspoon ground cumin
- 1 teaspoon paprika
- 1/2 teaspoon garlic powder
- 1/2 teaspoon onion powder
- 1/4 teaspoon cayenne pepper (adjust to taste)
- Salt to taste
- Fresh cilantro for garnish (optional)

INSTRUCTIONS

1. Preheat the Oven: Preheat your oven to 400°F (200°C). A baking sheet can be lightly oiled or lined with parchment paper.

2. Prepare the Chickpeas: Pat dry the rinsed chickpeas using a clean kitchen towel or paper towels. Ensure they are as dry as possible; this helps in achieving crispiness.

3. Season the Chickpeas: In a mixing bowl, combine the dried chickpeas with olive oil, chili powder, ground cumin, paprika, garlic powder, onion powder, cayenne pepper, and a

pinch of salt. Stir until the spice mixture coats the chickpeas evenly.

4. Bake the Chickpeas: Spread the seasoned chickpeas onto the prepared baking sheet in a single layer. Bake in the preheated oven for about 25-30 minutes, stirring halfway through, until the chickpeas are crispy and golden brown.

5. Cool and Serve: Allow the taco-spiced chickpeas to cool slightly. Garnish with fresh cilantro if desired. Serve as a snack or as a topping for salads or bowls.

NUTRITION INFO:

Calories: 150-200, Carbohydrates: 20-25g, Fiber: 5-7g, Protein: 5-7g, Fat: 5-7g

3. Keto candied nuts

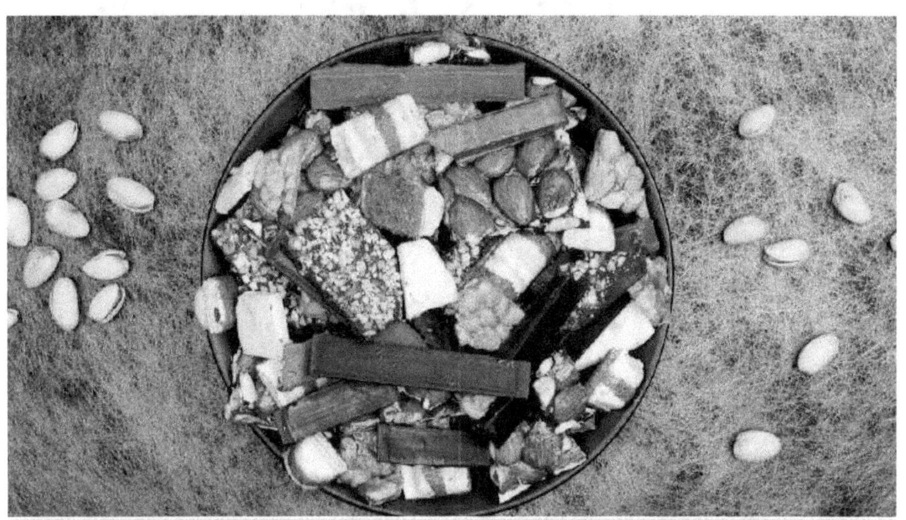

INGREDIENTS

- 2 cups mixed raw nuts (such as almonds, pecans, walnuts)
- 1/4 cup granulated monk fruit sweetener or erythritol
- 1 tablespoon butter or coconut oil, melted
- 1 teaspoon ground cinnamon
- 1/4 teaspoon salt
- 1/4 teaspoon vanilla extract

INSTRUCTIONS

1. Preheat the Oven: Preheat your oven to 300°F (150°C). Use a silicone baking mat or line a baking sheet with parchment paper.

2. Prepare the Nuts: In a mixing bowl, combine the mixed raw nuts with melted butter or coconut oil. Shake until the nuts are coated all over.

3. Create the Sweet Coating: In a separate bowl, mix the granulated monk fruit sweetener or erythritol, ground cinnamon, salt, and vanilla extract. Stir until well combined.

4. Coat the Nuts: Sprinkle the sweetener and spice mixture over the coated nuts. Toss well until the nuts are evenly coated with the sweet-spicy mix.

5. Bake the Nuts: Spread the coated nuts onto the prepared baking sheet in a single layer. Bake in the preheated oven for about 20-25 minutes, stirring halfway through, until the nuts are golden and fragrant.

6. Cool and Store: Remove the nuts from the oven and let them cool completely on the baking sheet. Place them in an airtight container to keep after they have cooled.

NUTRITION INFO:

Calories: 180-200, Carbohydrates: 5-7g, Fiber: 2-3g, Protein: 4-6g, Fat: 15-18g

4. Apple cinnamon bagels

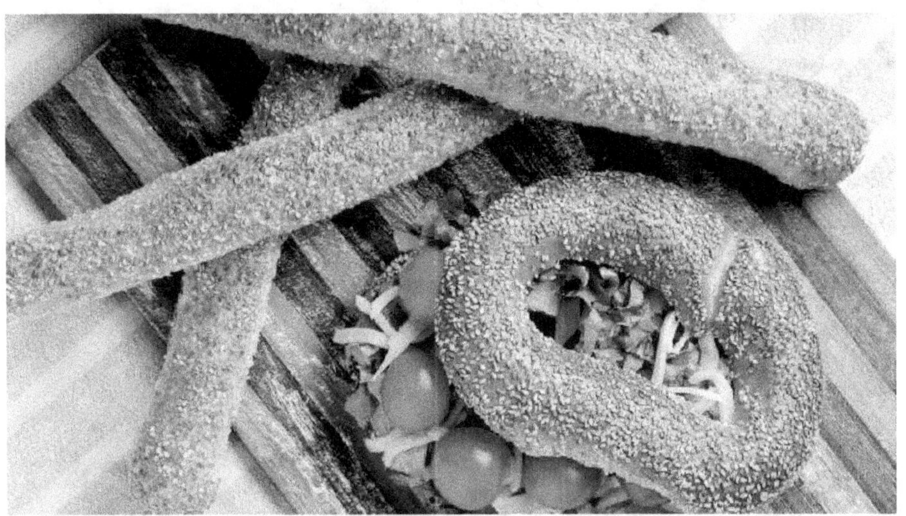

INGREDIENTS

- 1 cup almond flour
- 1/4 cup coconut flour
- 2 tablespoons ground flaxseed meal
- 1 teaspoon baking powder
- 1 teaspoon ground cinnamon
- Pinch of salt
- 2 large eggs
- 1/4 cup unsweetened applesauce
- 2 tablespoons melted coconut oil or butter
- 1 teaspoon vanilla extract

INSTRUCTIONS

1. Preheat the Oven: Preheat your oven to 350°F (175°C). Get a baking sheet ready and prepare it with silicone baking mats or parchment paper.

2. Prepare the Batter: In a mixing bowl, combine the almond flour, coconut flour, ground flaxseed meal, baking powder, ground cinnamon, and a pinch of salt. Mix well

3. Add Wet Ingredients: Add the eggs, unsweetened applesauce, melted coconut oil or butter, and vanilla extract to the dry

- 1 small apple, peeled and diced
- Optional: 1-2 tablespoons granulated sweetener of choice (such as monk fruit sweetener)

ingredients. Mix until a dough forms.

4. Fold in Apples: Gently fold in the diced apple pieces into the dough. If desired, add granulated sweetener to the dough for additional sweetness.

5. Shape Bagels: Divide the dough into equal portions and shape them into bagel rounds. You can use a donut or bagel mold if available or simply form them by hand.

6. Bake: Place the shaped bagels onto the prepared baking sheet. Bake in the preheated oven for about 20-25 minutes or until golden brown and cooked through.

7. Cool and Serve: Allow the bagels to cool on a wire rack before serving.

NUTRITION INFO:

Calories: 150-180, Carbohydrates: 8-10g, Fiber: 3-4g, Protein: 5-7g, Fat: 10-12g

Chapter 6: Recipes

SOME BAKED PRODUCTS WITH LOW GLYCEMIC LOAD

1. Whole Wheat Banana Bread

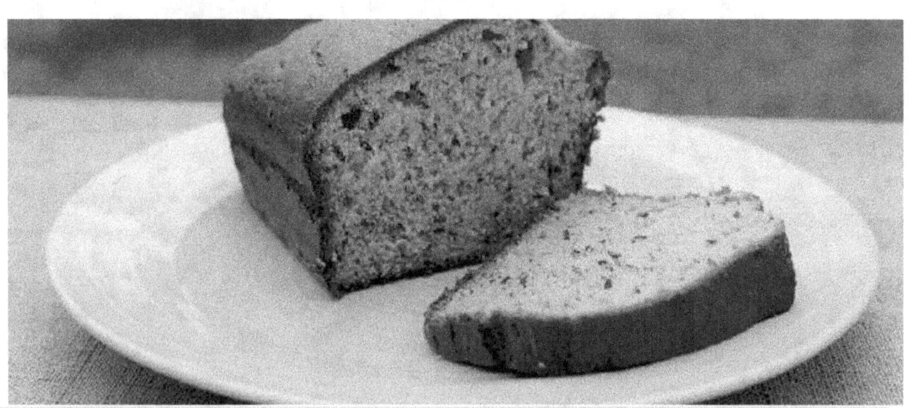

INGREDIENTS

-Whole wheat flour

-ripe bananas

-eggs

-Greek yogurt

-honey

-baking soda

-cinnamon

INSTRUCTIONS

1. Mix dry ingredients, then add mashed bananas, eggs, yogurt, and honey.
2. Bake at 350°F (175°C) for 50-60 mins.

NUTRITION INFO:

Fat: 10%, Protein: 15%, Carbs: 75%, Total Calories: ~150

2. Almond Flour Blueberry Muffins

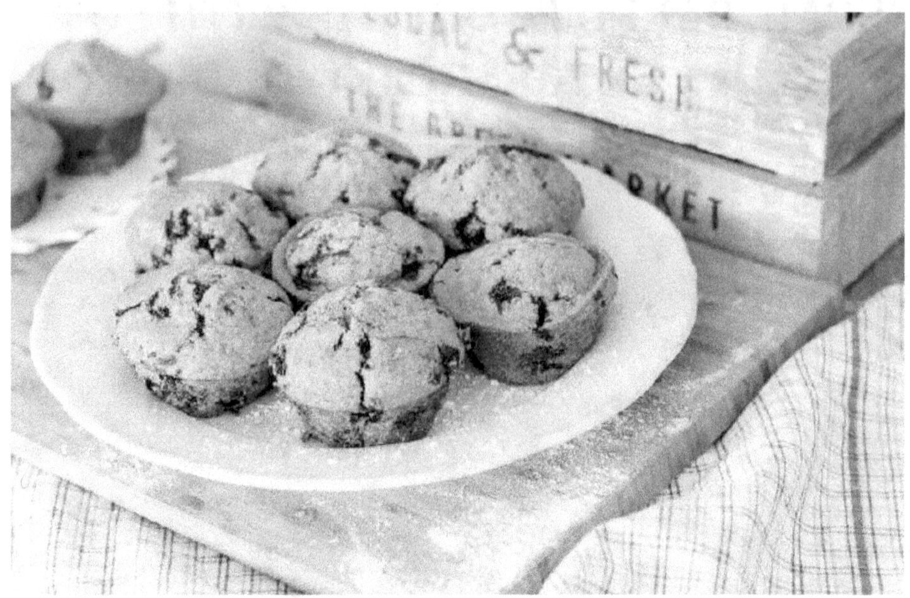

INGREDIENTS

- Almond flour
- eggs
- blueberries
- honey
- baking powder
- vanilla extract.

INSTRUCTIONS

1. Combine wet ingredients
2. add dry ingredients
3. fold in blueberries
4. bake at 350°F (175°C) for 20-25 mins.

NUTRITION INFO:

Fat: 60%, Protein: 15%, Carbs: 25%, Total Calories: ~200

3. Oatmeal Raisin Cookies

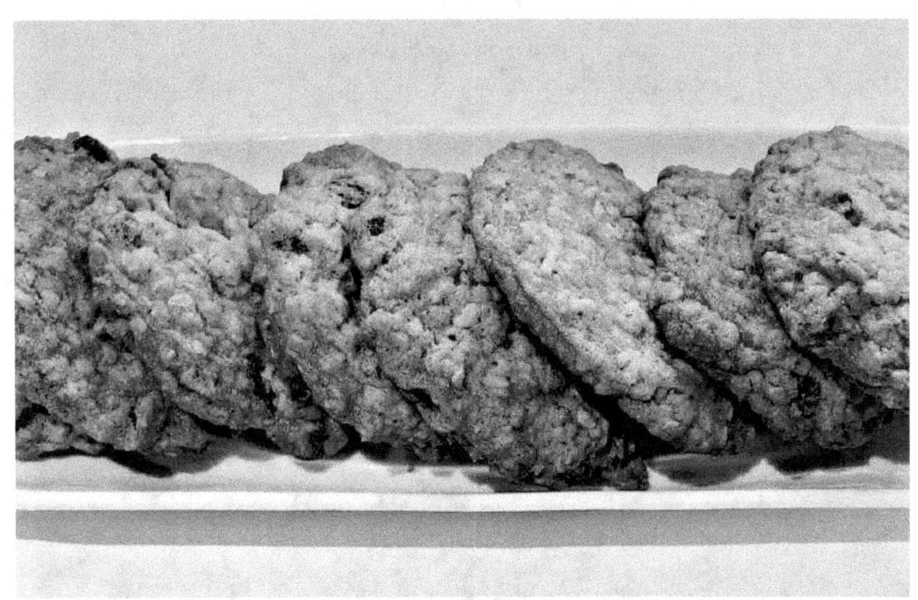

INGREDIENTS

-Rolled oats
-whole wheat flour
-raisins
-coconut oil
-honey
eggs
-cinnamon.

INSTRUCTIONS

1. Mix dry ingredients
2. add wet ingredients
3. shape into cookies
4. bake at 350°F (175°C) for 12-15 mins.

NUTRITION INFO:

Fat: 25%, Protein: 10%, Carbs: 65%, Total Calories: ~120

4. Pumpkin Spice Loaf

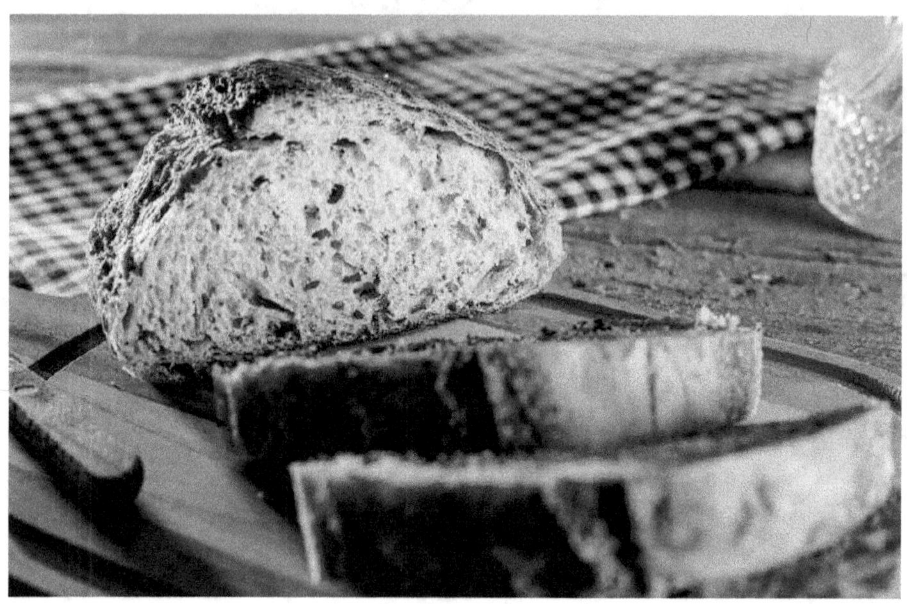

INGREDIENTS

-Pumpkin puree

-almond flour

-eggs

-maple syrup

-baking soda

-pumpkin spice.

INSTRUCTIONS

1. Mix ingredients
2. pour into a loaf pan
3. bake at 350°F (175°C) for 50-60 mins.

NUTRITION INFO:

Fat: 30%, Protein: 15%, Carbs: 55%, Total Calories: ~180

5. Coconut Flour Zucchini Bread

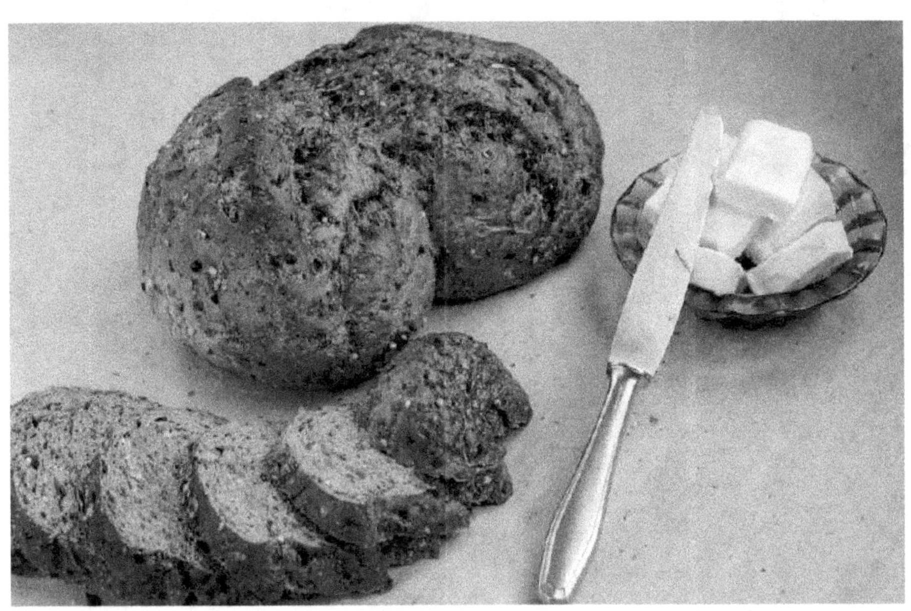

INGREDIENTS

-Coconut flour
-grated zucchini
-eggs
-Honey
-coconut oil
-baking soda
-cinnamon.

INSTRUCTIONS

1. Mix wet ingredients
2. fold in dry ingredients and zucchini
3. bake at 350°F (175°C) for 45-50 mins.

NUTRITION INFO:

Fat: 40%, Protein: 15%, Carbs: 45%, Total Calories: ~160

6. Apple Cinnamon Baked Oatmeal

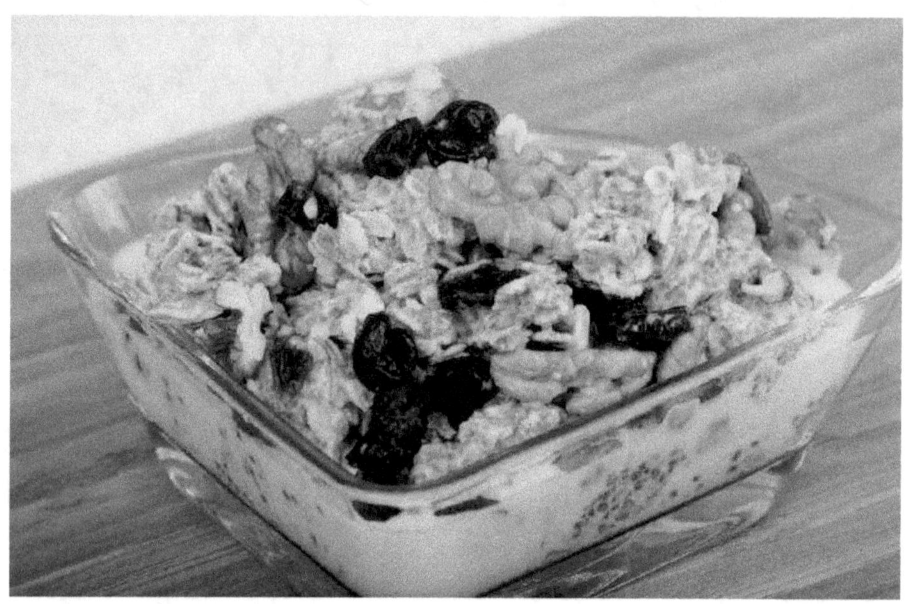

INGREDIENTS

- Rolled oats
- diced apples
- almond milk
- eggs
- honey
- cinnamon.

INSTRUCTIONS

1. Mix ingredients
2. pour into a baking dish
3. Bake at 350°F (175°C) for 25-30 mins.

NUTRITION INFO:

Fat: 20%, Protein: 15%, Carbs: 65%, Total Calories: ~180

7. Buckwheat Pancakes

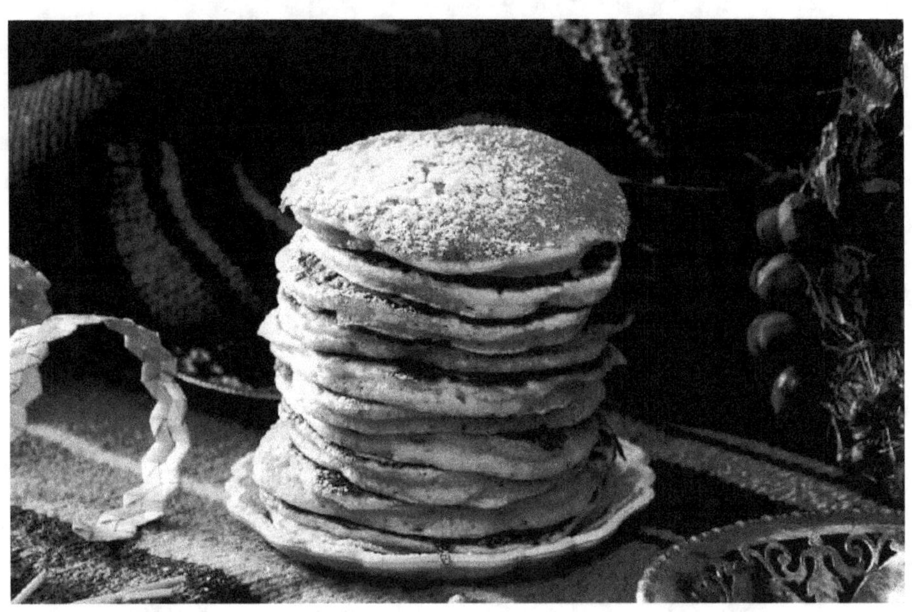

INGREDIENTS

-Buckwheat flour

-eggs

-almond milk

-baking powder

-honey.

INSTRUCTIONS

1. Mix ingredients
2. Cook pancakes on a skillet
3. flipping once bubbles form.

NUTRITION INFO:

Fat: 15%, Protein: 10%, Carbs: 75%, Total Calories: ~120

8. Lemon Poppy Seed Muffins

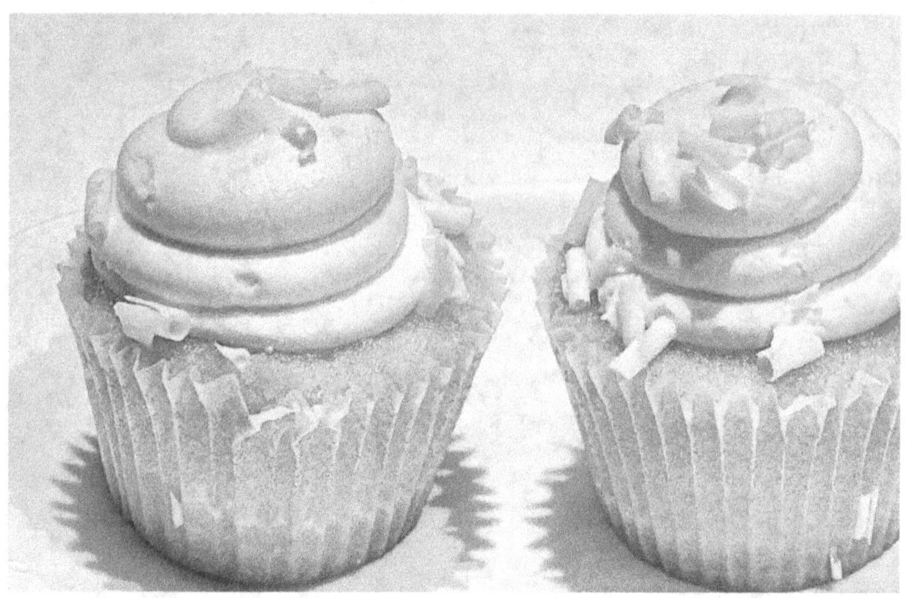

INGREDIENTS

- -Whole wheat flour
- -poppy seeds
- -lemon zest
- -Greek yogurt
- -honey, eggs
- -baking powder.

INSTRUCTIONS

1. Mix ingredients
2. bake at 350°F (175°C) for 20-25 mins.

NUTRITION INFO:

Fat: 20%, Protein: 15%, Carbs: 65%, Total Calories: ~150

9. Spelt Flour Pizza Dough

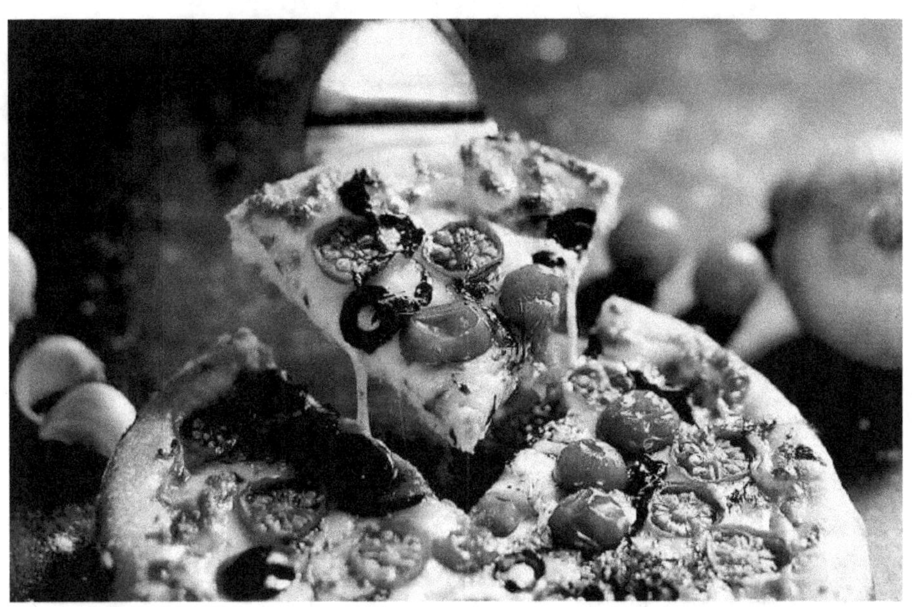

INGREDIENTS

-Spelt flour
-yeast, water
-olive oil
honey.

INSTRUCTIONS

1. Mix ingredients
2. let dough rise
3. roll out, add toppings
4. bake at 450°F (230°C) for 12-15 mins.

NUTRITION INFO:

Fat: 10%, Protein: 15%, Carbs: 75%, Total Calories: ~140

10. Sweet Potato Brownies

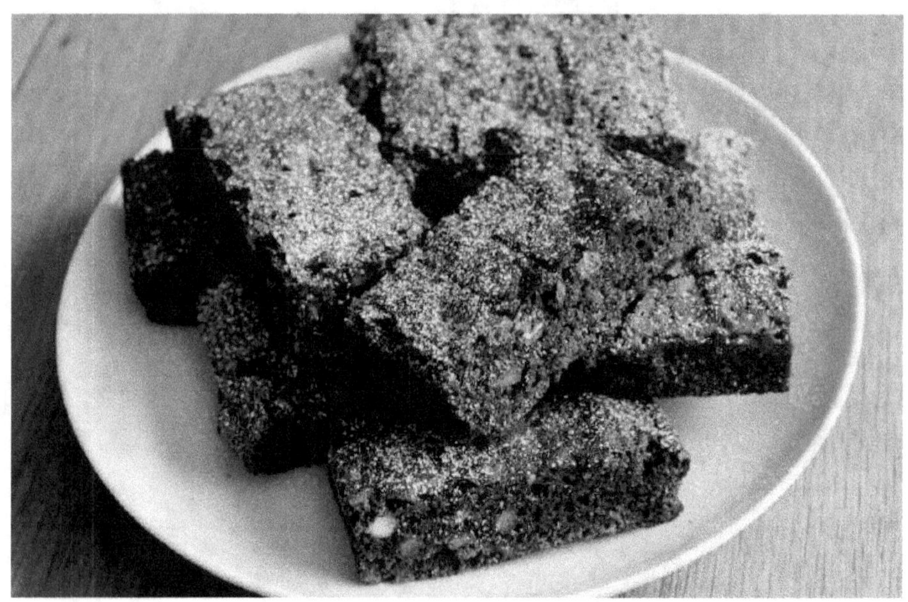

INGREDIENTS

-Sweet potatoes
-almond flour
-cocoa powder
-Honey
-eggs
-baking soda.

INSTRUCTIONS

1. Blend sweet potatoes
2. mix ingredients
3. Bake at 350°F (175°C) for 25-30 mins.

NUTRITION INFO:

Fat: 35%, Protein: 10%, Carbs: 55%, Total Calories: ~160

2 vegetable and vegetable products
1. Spinach salad

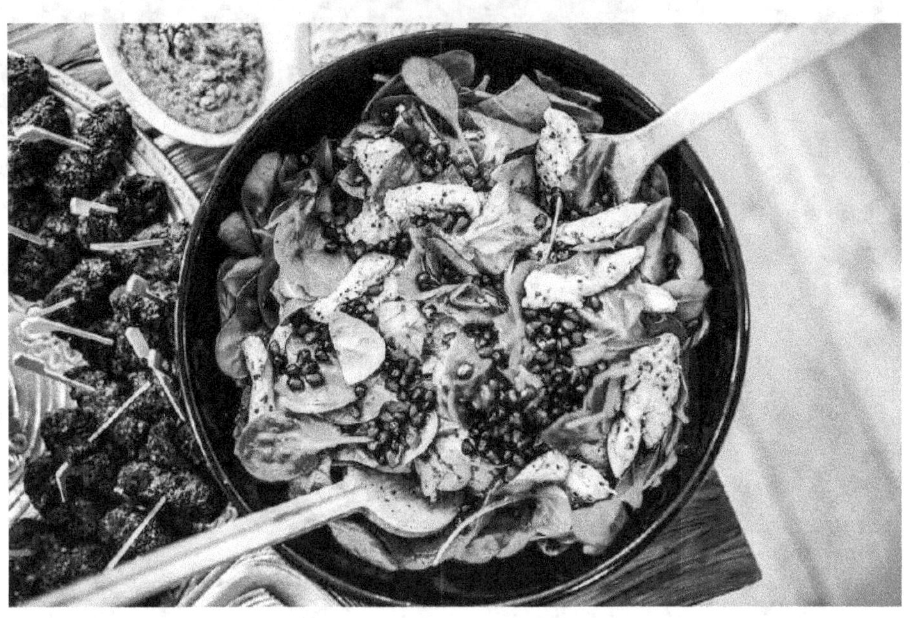

INGREDIENTS

-Fresh spinach leaves

-cherry tomatoes

-red onion

-feta cheese

-olive oil

-balsamic vinegar.

INSTRUCTIONS

1. Toss spinach with chopped tomatoes, onion, and feta.

2. Pour some balsamic vinegar and olive oil over it.

NUTRITION INFO:

Fat: 60%, Protein: 20%, Carbs: 20%, Total Calories: ~100

2. Garlic Roasted Broccoli

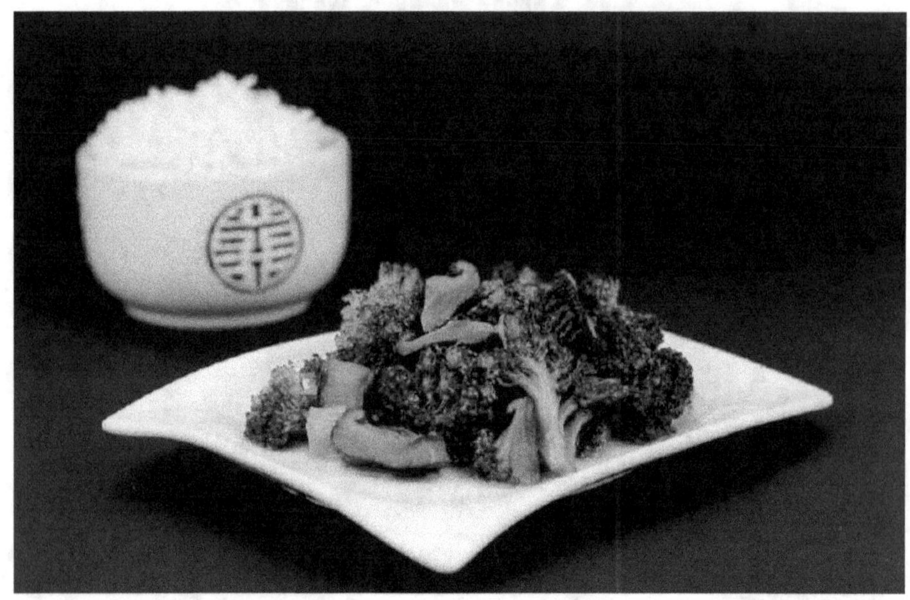

INGREDIENTS

-Broccoli florets
-minced garlic
-olive oil
-salt
-pepper.

INSTRUCTIONS

1. Toss broccoli with garlic, olive oil, salt, and pepper.
2. Roast at 400°F (200°C) for 20-25 mins.

NUTRITION INFO:

Fat: 50%, Protein: 25%, Carbs: 25%, Total Calories: ~50

3. Stuffed Bell Peppers

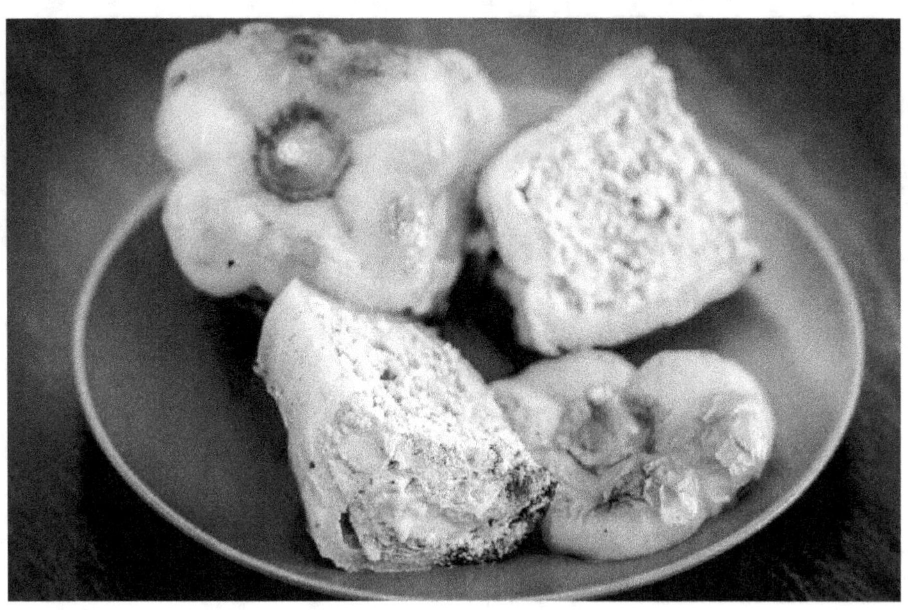

INGREDIENTS

-Bell peppers

-quinoa

-black beans

-corn

-onions

-tomatoes

-spices.

INSTRUCTIONS

1. Stuff halved peppers with cooked quinoa, beans, corn, onions, tomatoes, and spices.
2. Bake at 375°F (190°C) for 25-30 mins.

NUTRITION INFO:

Fat: 20%, Protein: 30%, Carbs: 50%, Total Calories: ~200

4. Zucchini Noodles (Zoodles)

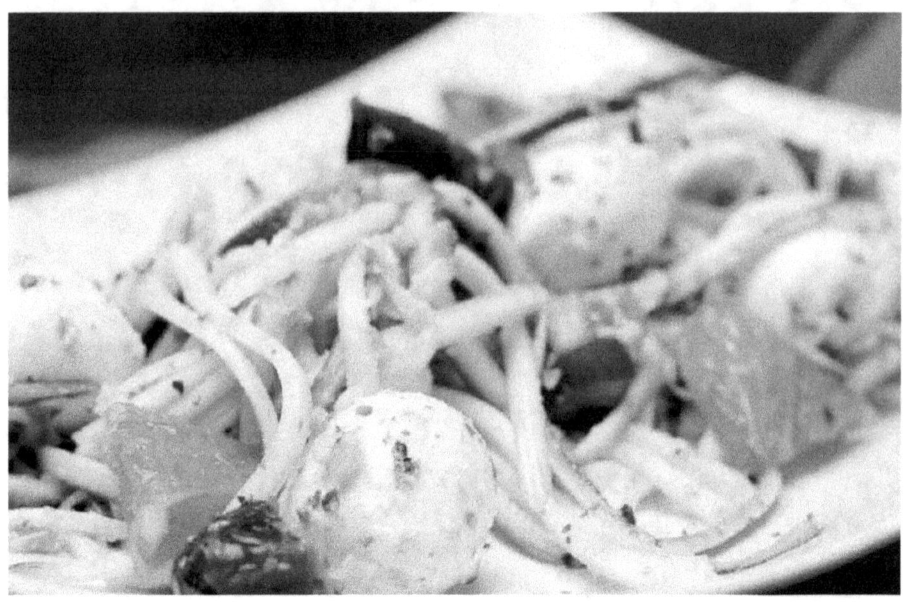

INGREDIENTS

- -Zucchini
- -olive oil
- -garlic
- -salt
- -pepper.

INSTRUCTIONS

1. Spiralize zucchini into noodles.
2. Sauté with garlic, olive oil, salt, and pepper.

NUTRITION INFO:

Fat: 70%, Protein: 15%, Carbs: 15%, Total Calories: ~30

5. Cauliflower Rice

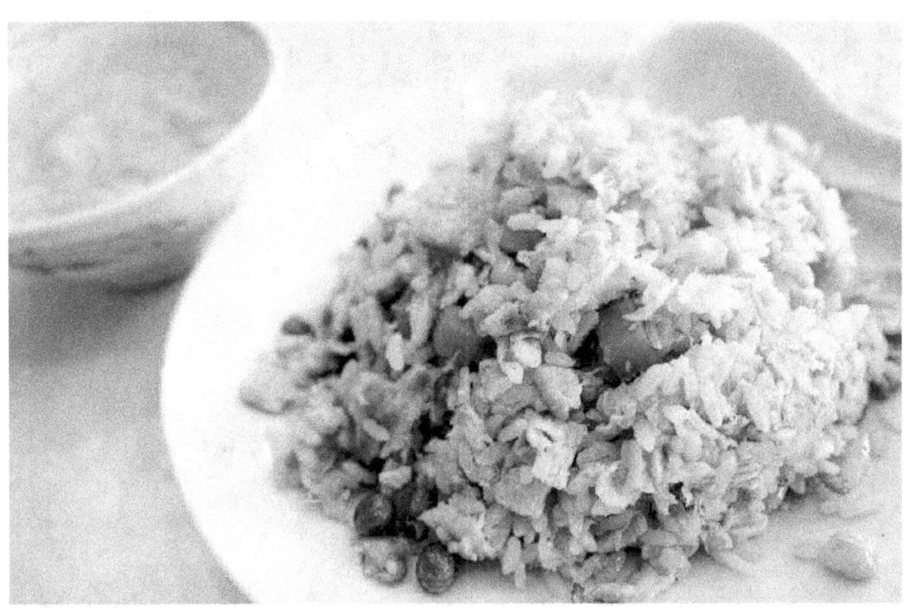

INGREDIENTS

- Pumpkin puree
- almond flour
- eggs
- maple syrup
- baking soda
- pumpkin spice.

INSTRUCTIONS

1. Mix ingredients
2. pour into a loaf pan
3. bake at 350°F (175°C) for 50-60 mins.

NUTRITION INFO:

Fat: 60%, Protein: 20%, Carbs: 20%, Total Calories: ~50

6. Grilled Asparagus

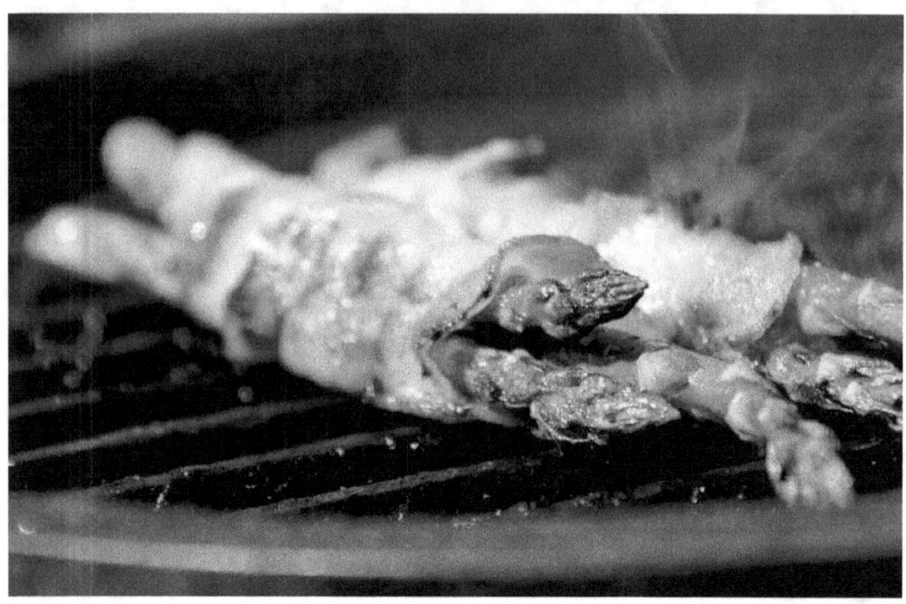

INGREDIENTS

-Asparagus spears

-olive oil

-lemon juice

-salt

-pepper.

INSTRUCTIONS

1. Toss asparagus with olive oil, lemon juice, salt, and pepper.
2. Grill for 5-7 mins.

NUTRITION INFO:

Fat: 70%, Protein: 20%, Carbs: 10%, Total Calories: ~40

7. Eggplant Parmesan

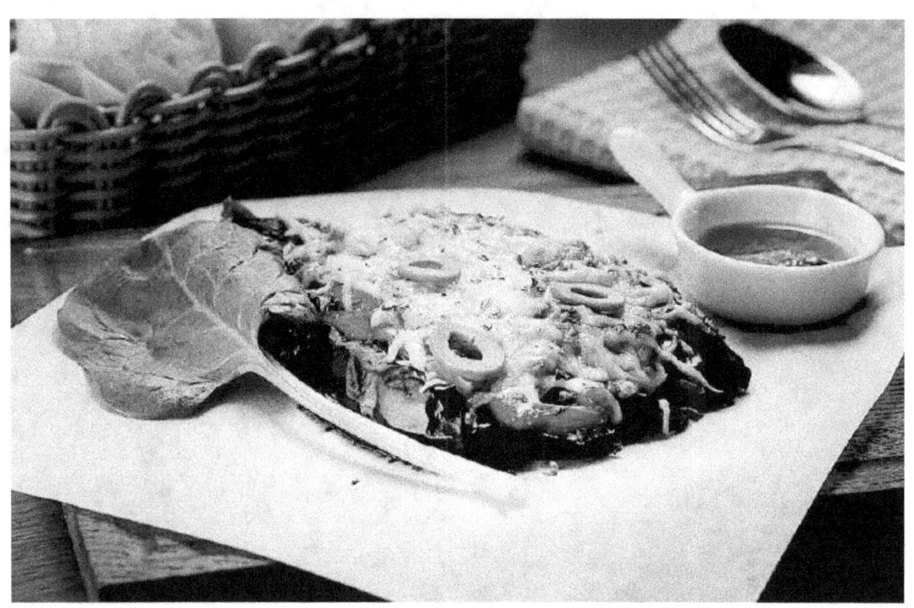

INGREDIENTS

-Eggplant slices
-breadcrumbs
-marinara sauce
-mozzarella cheese
-Parmesan cheese.

INSTRUCTIONS

1. Coat eggplant in breadcrumbs, bake until golden.
2. Layer with marinara and cheeses, bake until bubbly.

NUTRITION INFO:

Fat: 40%, Protein: 25%, Carbs: 35%, Total Calories: ~150

8. Cabbage Stir-Fry

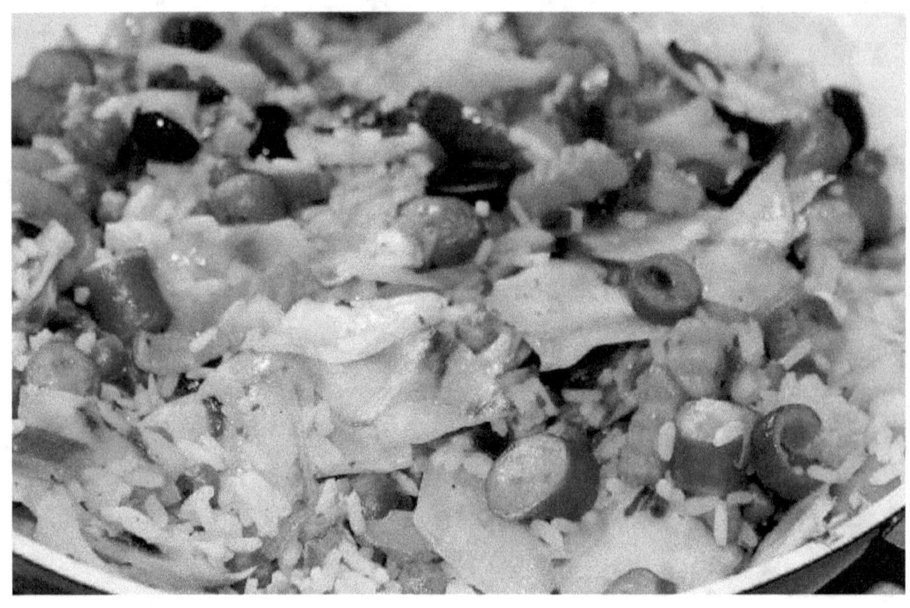

INGREDIENTS

-Sliced cabbage

-carrots

-bell peppers

-soy sauce

-ginger, garlic.

INSTRUCTIONS

1. Stir-fry vegetables with soy sauce, ginger, and garlic until tender.

NUTRITION INFO:

Fat: 25%, Protein: 10%, Carbs: 65%, Total Calories: ~50

9. Kale Chips

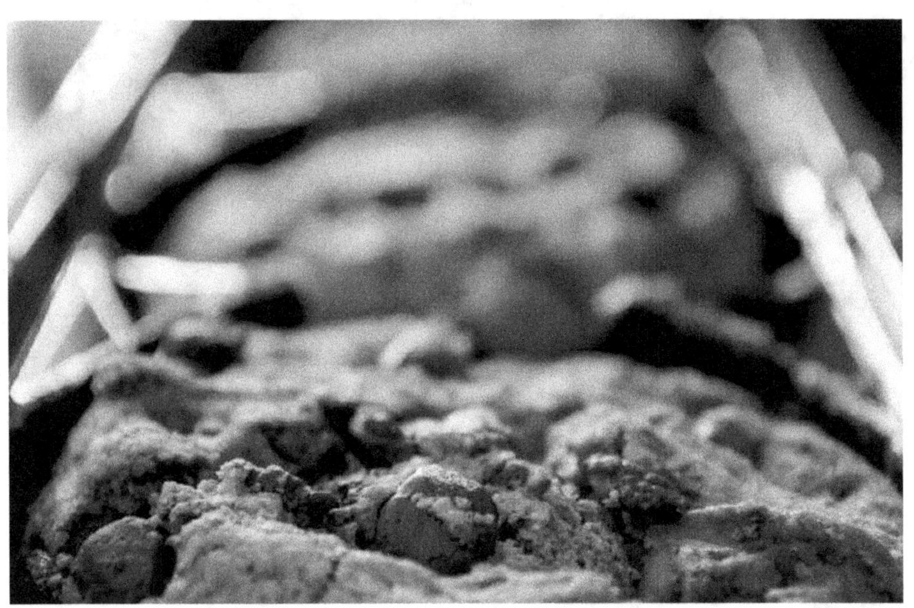

INGREDIENTS

-Kale leaves
-olive oil
-salt
-nutritional yeast
(optional).

INSTRUCTIONS

1. Massage kale with oil, sprinkle with salt and nutritional yeast.
2. Bake at 300°F (150°C) for 10-15 mins.

NUTRITION INFO:

Fat: 60%, Protein: 20%, Carbs: 20%, Total Calories: ~50

10. Caprese Salad

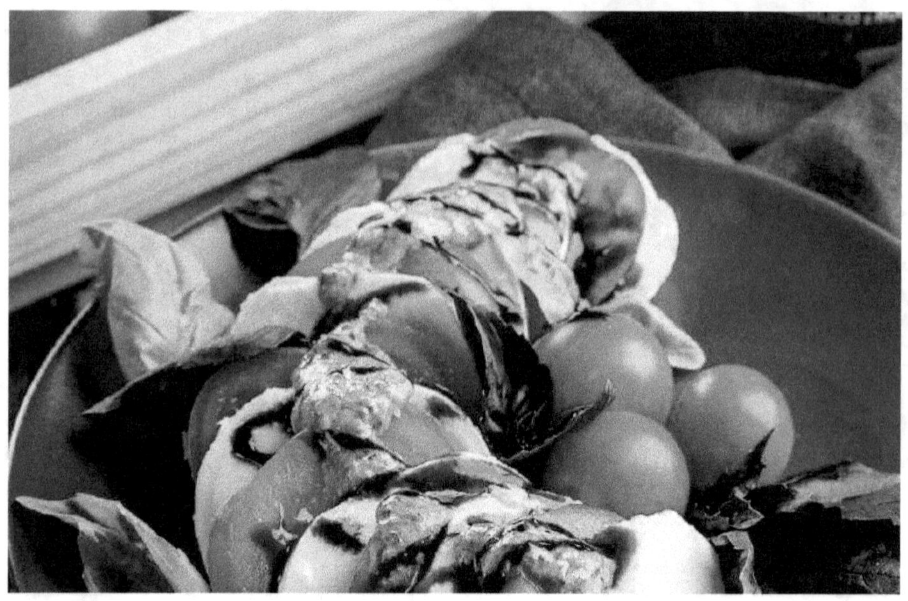

INGREDIENTS

- Tomato slices
- fresh mozzarella
- basil leaves
- olive oil
- balsamic glaze.

INSTRUCTIONS

1. Layer tomatoes, mozzarella, and basil. Brush with a balsamic glaze and olive oil.

NUTRITION INFO:

Fat: 55%, Protein: 30%, Carbs: 15%, Total Calories: ~100

Fruit and fruit products
1. Berry Smoothie

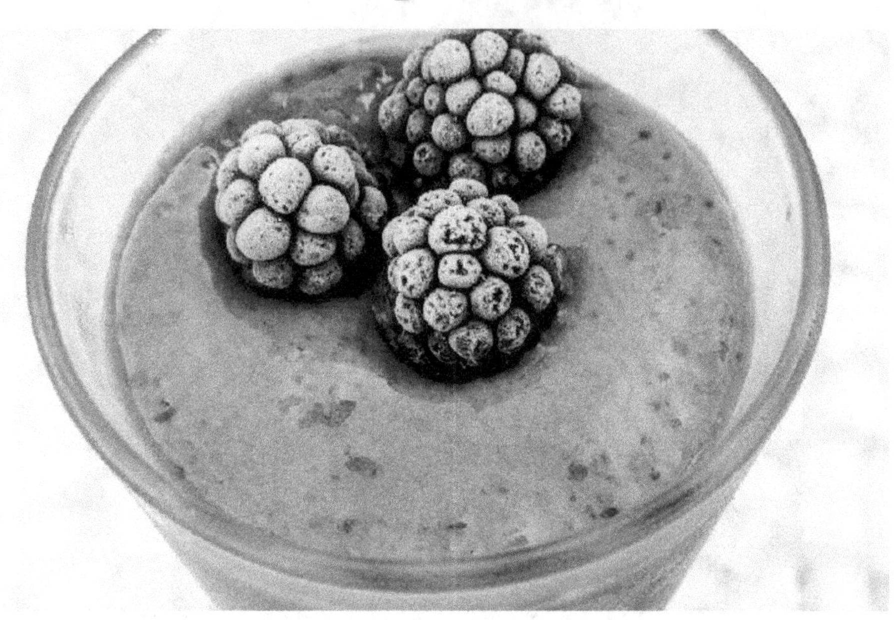

INGREDIENTS

- Mixed berries
- Greek yogurt
- almond milk
- honey.

INSTRUCTIONS

1. Blend berries, yogurt, almond milk, and honey until smooth.

NUTRITION INFO:

Fat: 10%, Protein: 15%, Carbs: 75%, Total Calories: ~100

2. Baked Apple Slices

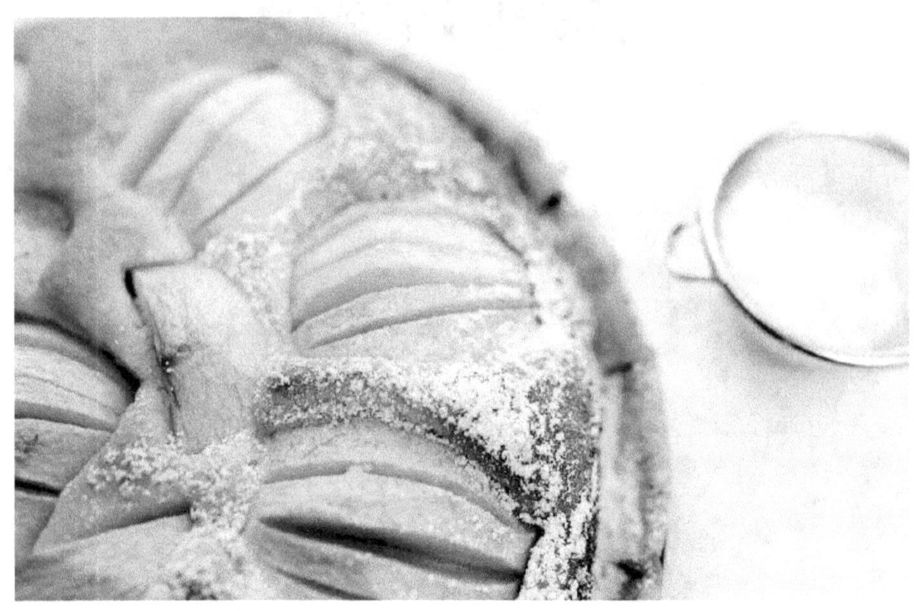

INGREDIENTS

-Apple slices
-cinnamon
-coconut oil.

INSTRUCTIONS

1. Toss apple slices with cinnamon and coconut oil.
2. Bake at 350°F (175°C) for 20-25 mins.

NUTRITION INFO:

Fat: 40%, Protein: 5%, Carbs: 55%, Total Calories: ~80

3. Poached Pears

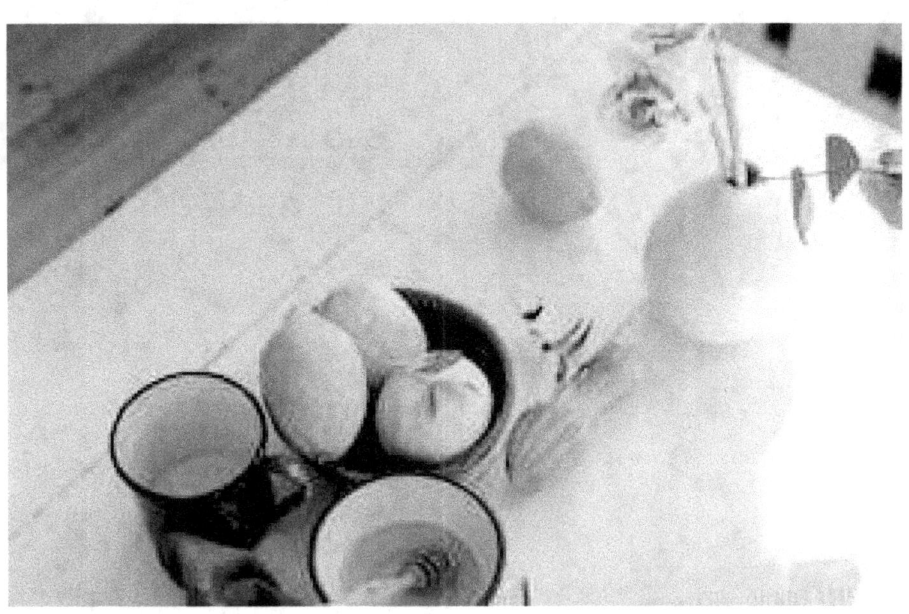

INGREDIENTS

- Pears
- water
- honey
- cinnamon.

INSTRUCTIONS

1. Simmer pears in water, honey, and cinnamon until tender.

NUTRITION INFO:

Fat: 5%, Protein: 5%, Carbs: 90%, Total Calories: ~90

4. Cherry Chia Seed Pudding

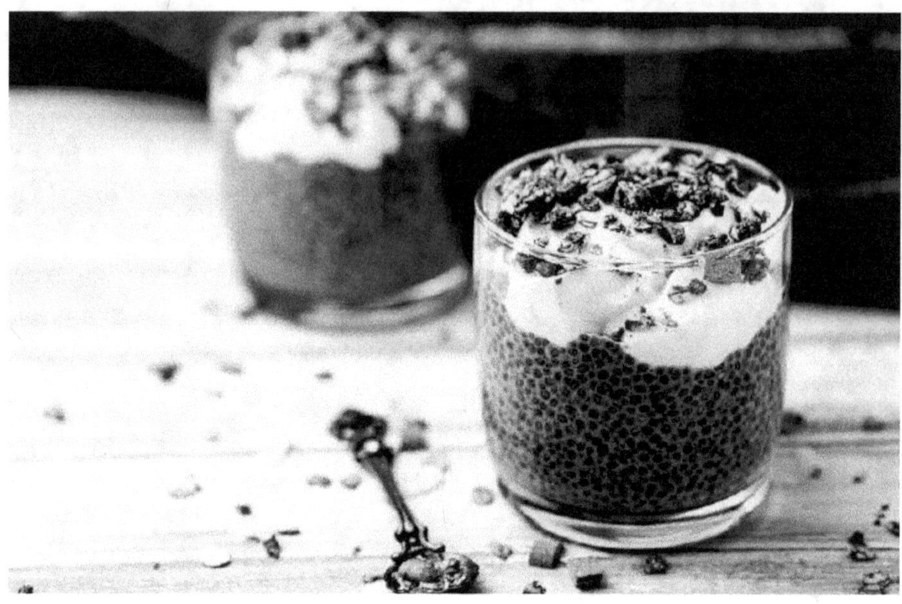

INGREDIENTS

-Cherries

-chia seeds

-almond milk

-honey.

INSTRUCTIONS

1. Blend cherries and almond milk, mix with chia seeds and honey, refrigerate overnight.

NUTRITION INFO:

Fat: 25%, Protein: 10%, Carbs: 65%, Total Calories: ~120

5. Grilled Apricots

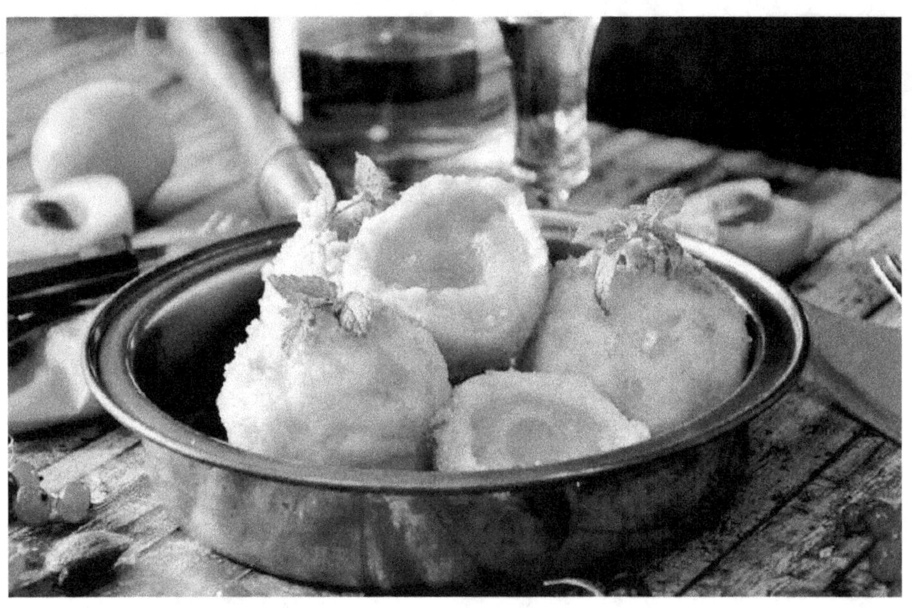

INGREDIENTS

-Halved apricots
-honey
-cinnamon.

INSTRUCTIONS

1. Grill apricots until slightly caramelized, drizzle with honey and sprinkle cinnamon.

NUTRITION INFO:

Fat: 5%, Protein: 5%, Carbs: 90%, Total Calories: ~70

6. Kiwi and Yogurt Parfait

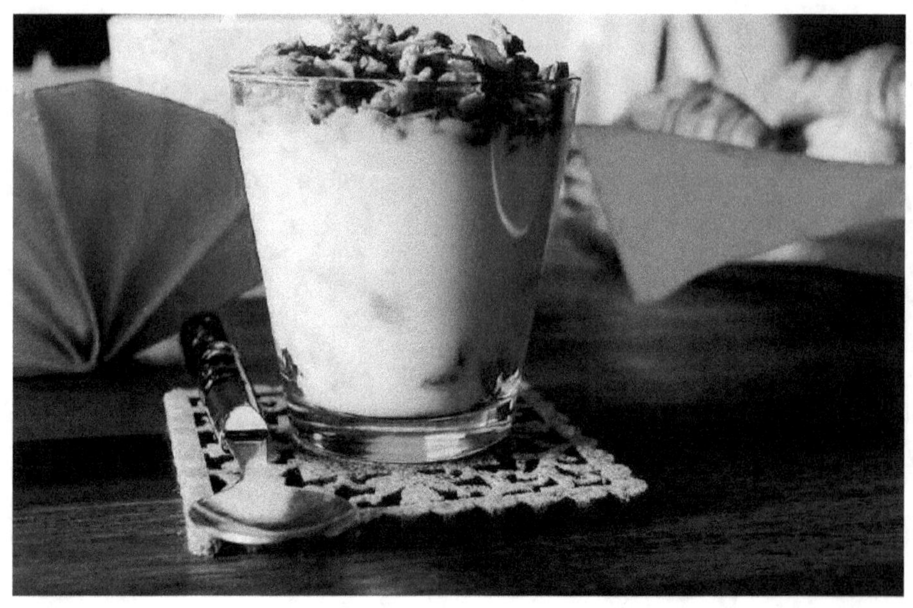

INGREDIENTS

-Sliced kiwi
-Greek yogurt
-granola.

INSTRUCTIONS

1. Layer kiwi slices, yogurt, and granola in a glass.

NUTRITION INFO:

Fat: 15%, Protein: 25%, Carbs: 60%, Total Calories: ~90

7. Orange Salad

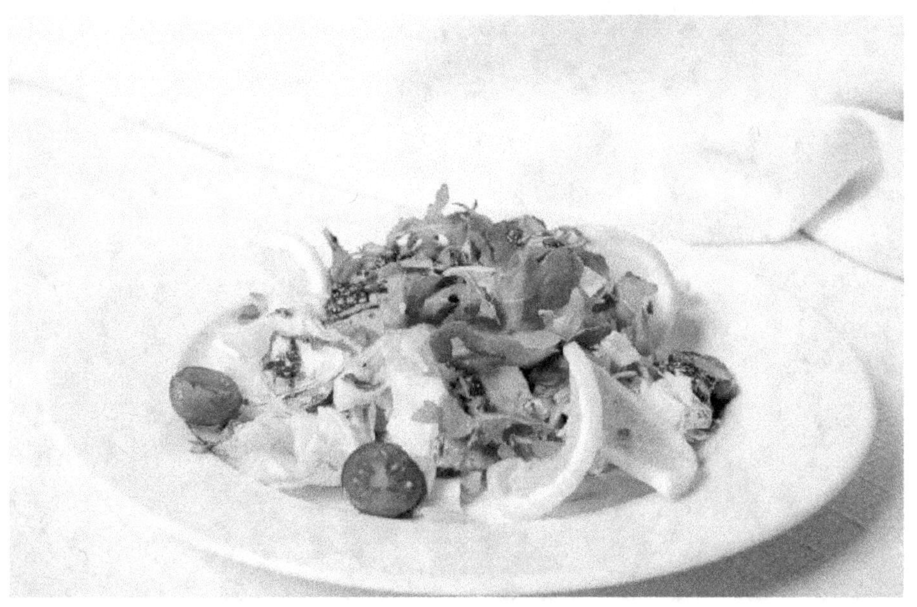

INGREDIENTS

-Orange slices
-mixed greens
-feta cheese
-balsamic vinaigrette.

INSTRUCTIONS

1. Toss orange slices with mixed greens, top with feta, and drizzle with vinaigrette.

NUTRITION INFO:

Fat: 40%, Protein: 10%, Carbs: 50%, Total Calories: ~70

8. Grilled Peaches with Yogurt

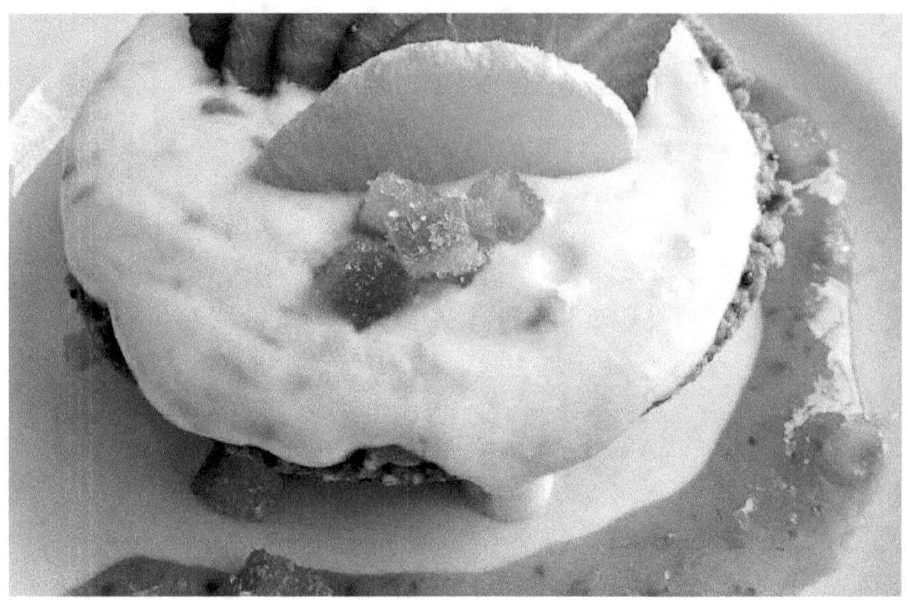

INGREDIENTS

-Halved peaches
-Greek yogurt
-honey.

INSTRUCTIONS

1. Grill peaches, serve with a dollop of yogurt and a drizzle of honey.

NUTRITION INFO:

Fat: 20%, Protein: 20%, Carbs: 60%, Total Calories: ~80

9. Plum Compote

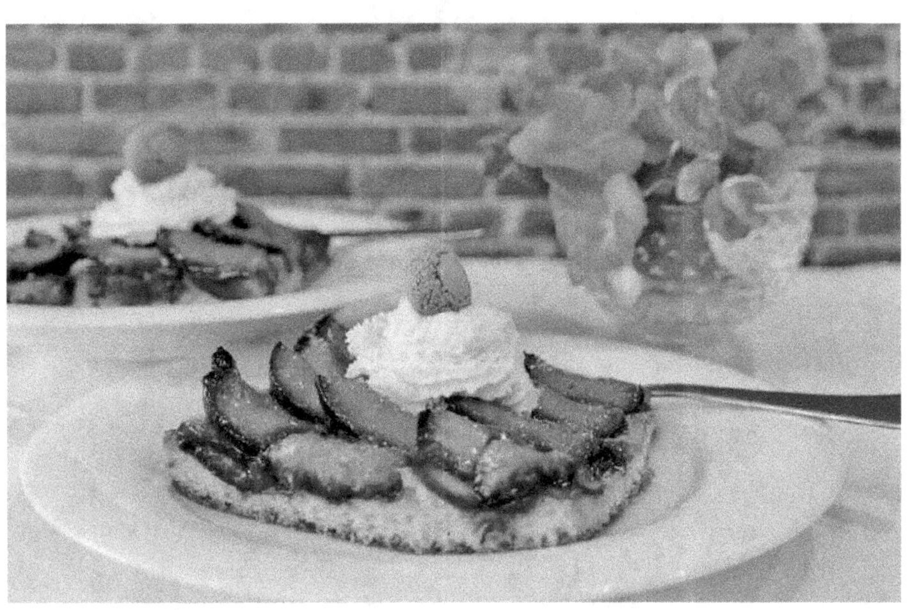

INGREDIENTS

-Sliced plums

-water, honey

-vanilla extract.

INSTRUCTIONS

1. Simmer plums in water, honey, and vanilla until softened.

NUTRITION INFO:

Fat: 5%, Protein: 5%, Carbs: 90%, Total Calories: ~70

10. Broiled Grapefruit

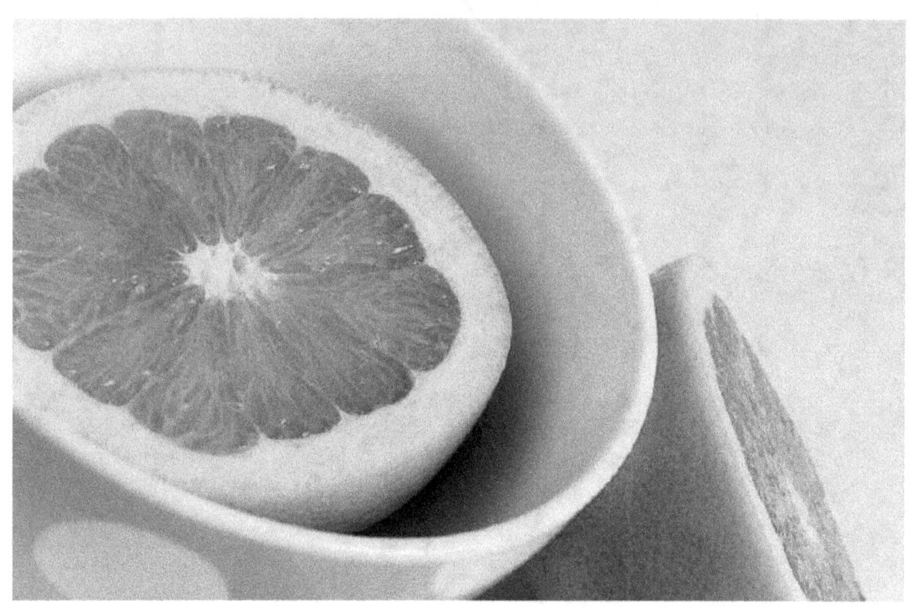

INGREDIENTS

-Grapefruit halves
-honey
-cinnamon.

INSTRUCTIONS

1. Broil grapefruit halves, drizzle with honey, and sprinkle cinnamon.

NUTRITION INFO:

Fat: 5%, Protein: 5%, Carbs: 90%, Total Calories: ~60

Grains and breakfast cereal
1. Quinoa Breakfast Bowl

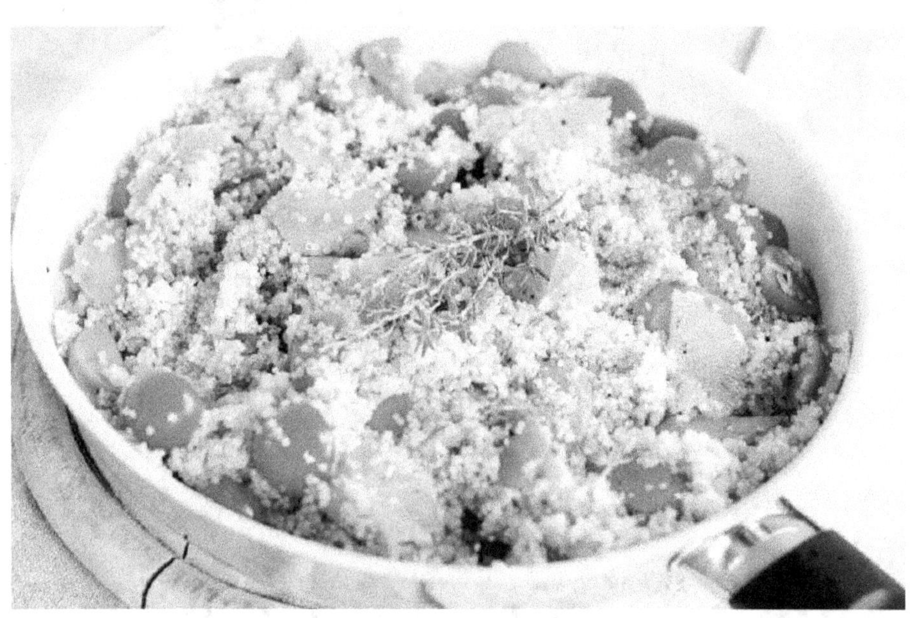

INGREDIENTS

-Cooked quinoa
-sliced bananas
-almond butter
-cinnamon.

INSTRUCTIONS

1. Mix quinoa with sliced bananas, top with almond butter and a sprinkle of cinnamon.

NUTRITION INFO:

Fat: 30%, Protein: 20%, Carbs: 50%, Total Calories: ~200

2. Overnight Oats

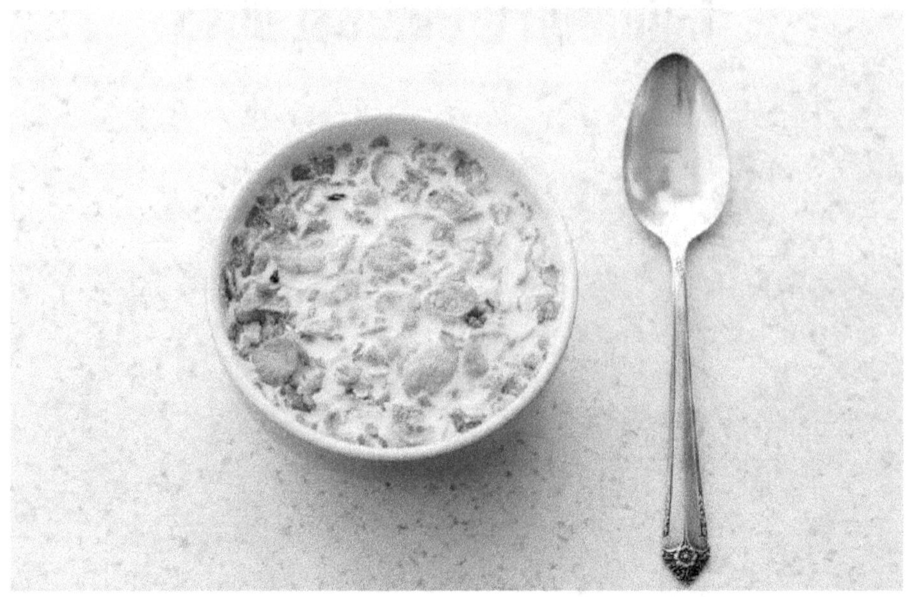

INGREDIENTS

-Rolled oats

-chia seeds

-almond milk

-mixed berries

-honey.

INSTRUCTIONS

1. Mix oats, chia seeds, almond milk, and honey in a jar.
2. Refrigerate overnight, top with berries before serving.

NUTRITION INFO:

Fat: 20%, Protein: 15%, Carbs: 65%, Total Calories: ~180

3. Barley Breakfast Porridge

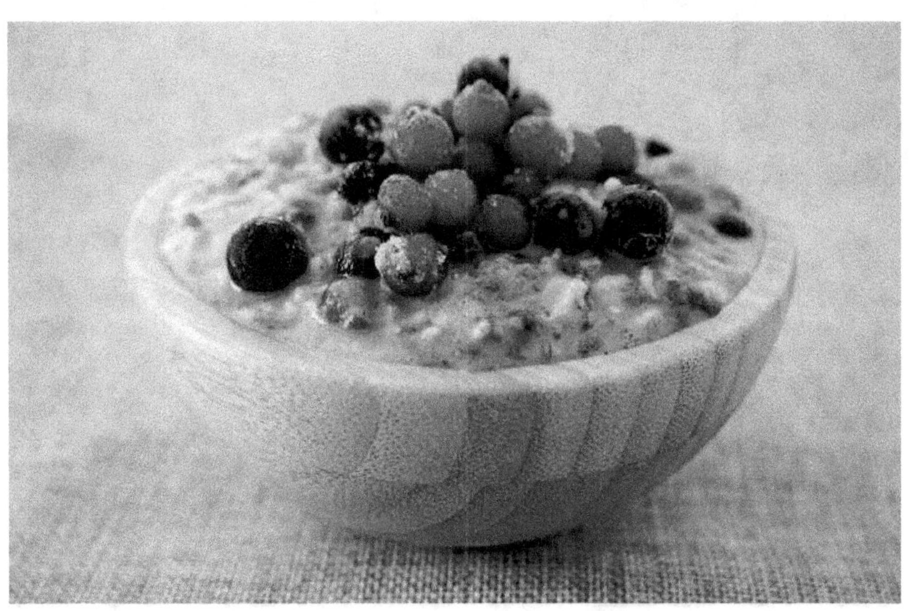

INGREDIENTS

-Cooked barley

-unsweetened almond milk

-diced apples

-nuts

-honey.

INSTRUCTIONS

1. Simmer barley in almond milk, add diced apples, nuts, and honey.

NUTRITION INFO:

Fat: 25%, Protein: 15%, Carbs: 60%, Total Calories: ~220

4. Brown Rice Breakfast Bowl

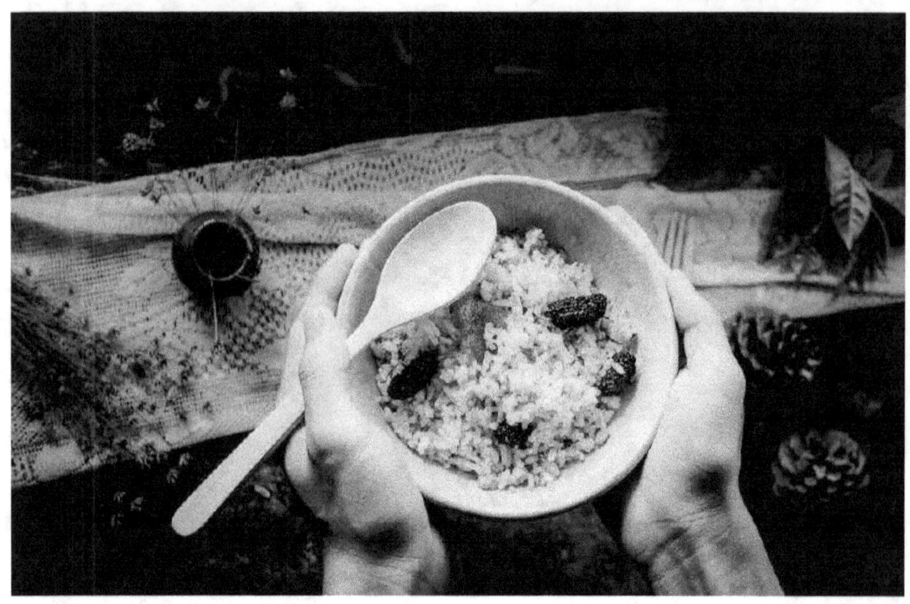

INGREDIENTS

-Cooked brown rice

-Greek yogurt

-mixed berries

-sliced almonds

-honey.

INSTRUCTIONS

1. Top brown rice with yogurt, berries, almonds, and a drizzle of honey.

NUTRITION INFO:

Fat: 20%, Protein: 15%, Carbs: 65%, Total Calories: ~190

5. Whole Grain Toast with Avocado

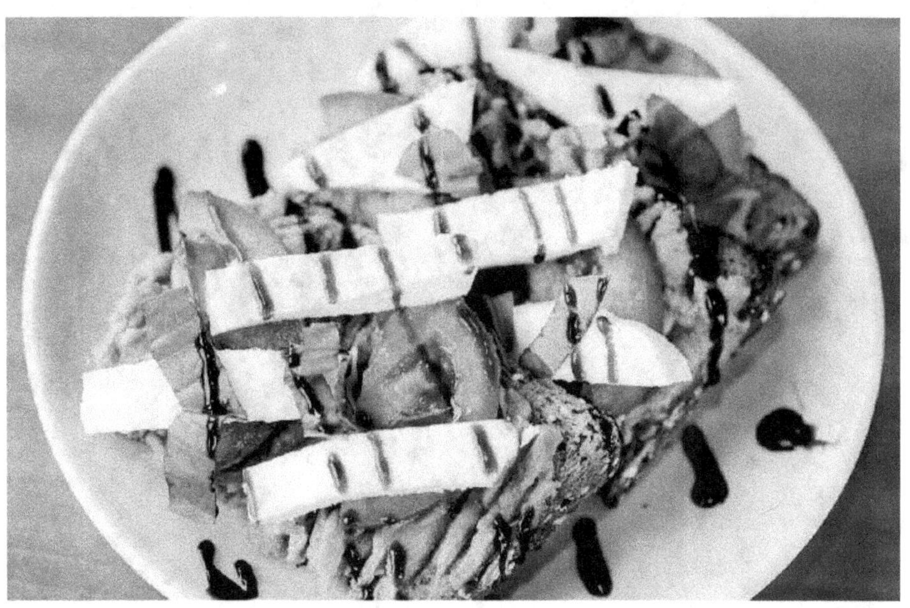

INGREDIENTS

-Whole grain bread slices

-mashed avocado

-sea salt

-red pepper flakes.

INSTRUCTIONS

1. Toast bread, spread avocado, sprinkle with salt and pepper flakes.

NUTRITION INFO:

Fat: 15%, Protein: 10%, Carbs: 75%, Total Calories: ~100

6. Millet Breakfast Porridge

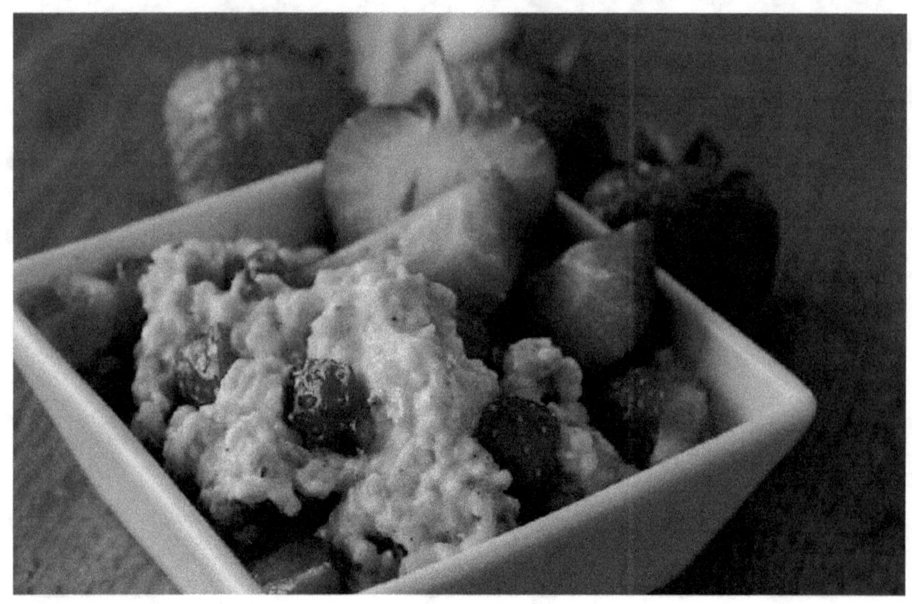

INGREDIENTS

-Cooked millet
-coconut milk
-sliced mango
-shredded coconut
-honey.

INSTRUCTIONS

1. Simmer millet in coconut milk, top with mango, shredded coconut, and honey.

NUTRITION INFO:

Fat: 30%, Protein: 10%, Carbs: 60%, Total Calories: ~210

7. Bulgur Breakfast Bowl

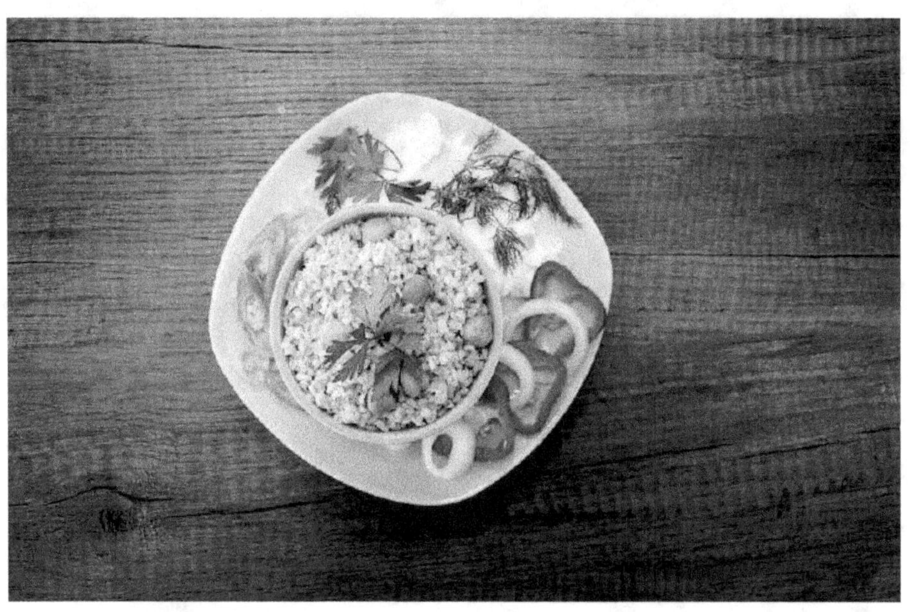

INGREDIENTS

-Cooked bulgur

-diced peaches

-Greek yogurt

-sliced almonds

-maple syrup.

INSTRUCTIONS

1. Mix bulgur with peaches, yogurt, almonds, and maple syrup.

NUTRITION INFO:

Fat: 20%, Protein: 15%, Carbs: 65%, Total Calories: ~180

8. Amaranth Breakfast Bowl

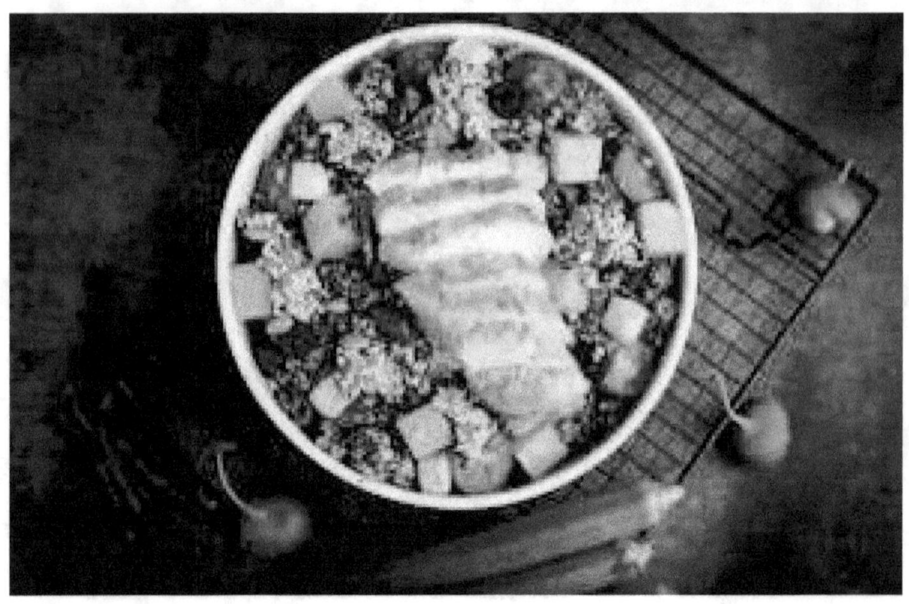

INGREDIENTS

-Cooked amaranth
-mixed berries
-sliced bananas
-almond butter
-honey.

INSTRUCTIONS

1. Mix amaranth with berries, bananas, almond butter, and honey.

NUTRITION INFO:

Fat: 25%, Protein: 15%, Carbs: 60%, Total Calories: ~180

Beef, lamb, veal, pork, and poultry
1. Grilled Chicken Skewers

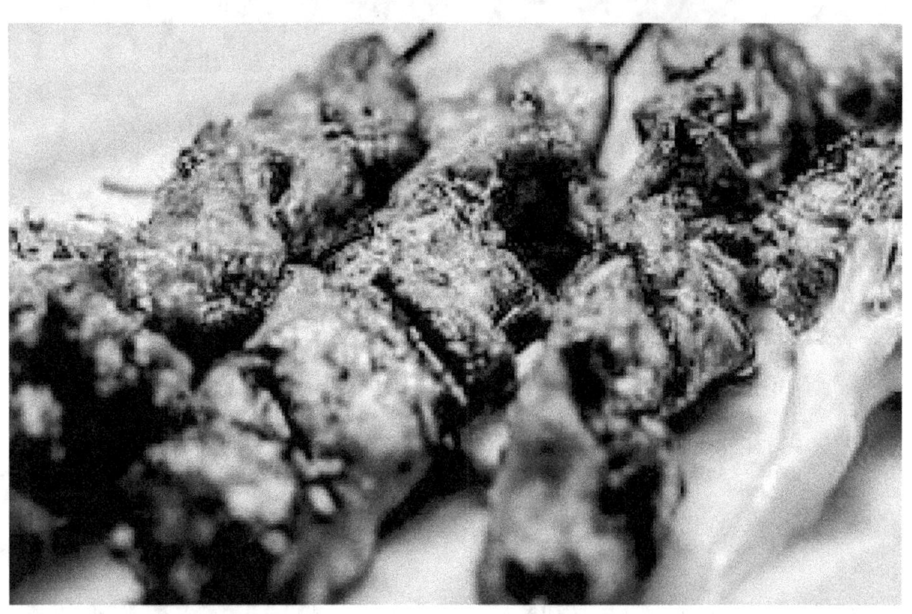

INGREDIENTS

-Chicken breast

-bell peppers

-onions

-olive oil

-garlic

-lemon juice

-herbs.

INSTRUCTIONS

1. Cube chicken, marinate in olive oil, garlic, lemon juice, herbs. Skewer with peppers and onions, grill until cooked.

NUTRITION INFO:

Fat: 15%, Protein: 65%, Carbs: 20%, Total Calories: ~180

2. Pork Tenderloin with Apple Compote

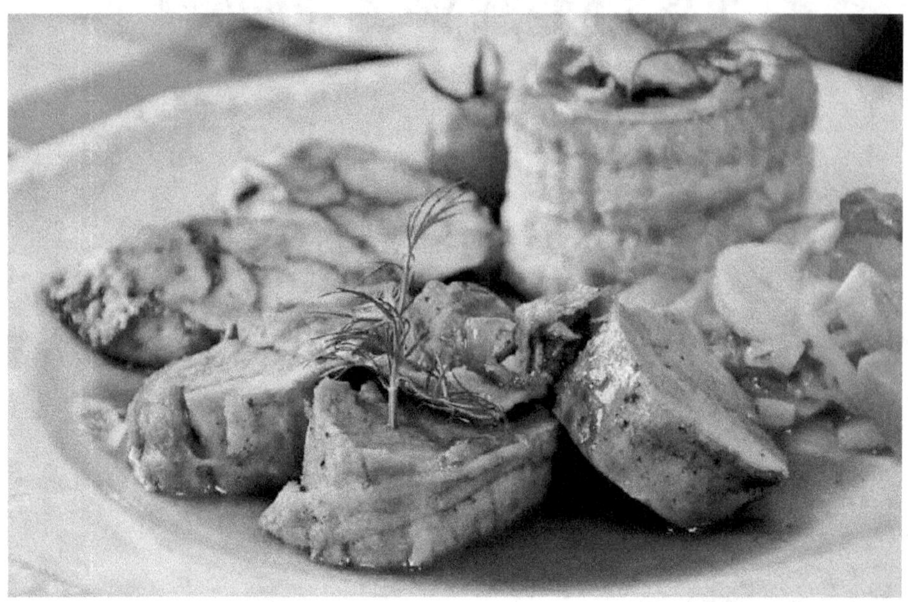

INGREDIENTS

- Pork tenderloin
- apples
- cinnamon
- honey.

INSTRUCTIONS

1. Roast pork, cook apples with cinnamon and honey until softened.
2. Serve over sliced pork.

NUTRITION INFO:

Fat: 25%, Protein: 60%, Carbs: 15%, Total Calories: ~160

3. Beef Stir-Fry

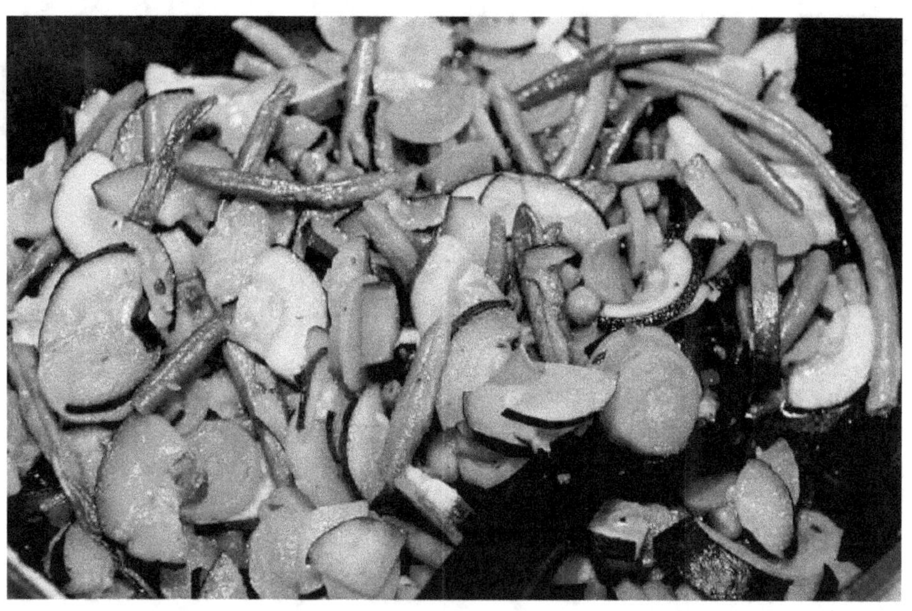

INGREDIENTS

-Lean beef strips
-broccoli
-bell peppers
-soy sauce
-ginger
-garlic.

INSTRUCTIONS

1. Stir-fry beef and vegetables with soy sauce, ginger, and garlic until cooked.

NUTRITION INFO:

Fat: 20%, Protein: 50%, Carbs: 30%, Total Calories: ~200

4. Veal Scallopini with Mushroom Sauce

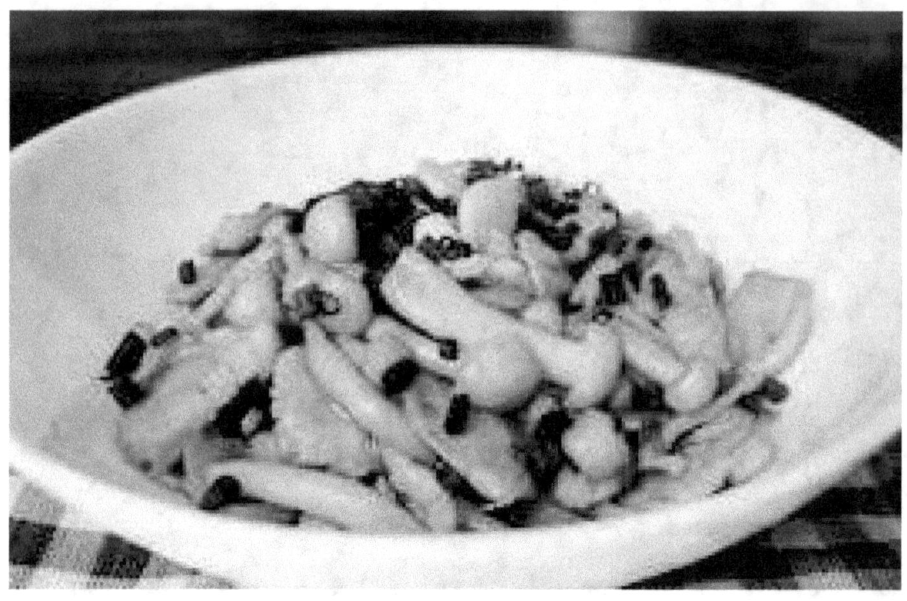

INGREDIENTS

-Pork tenderloin

-apples

--Veal scallopini

-mushrooms

-onions

-garlic

-chicken broth

-thyme.

INSTRUCTIONS

1. Sauté veal, cook mushrooms, onions, and garlic in broth. Serve veal with mushroom sauce.

NUTRITION INFO:

Fat: 30%, Protein: 55%, Carbs: 15%, Total Calories: ~190

5. Lamb Kebabs

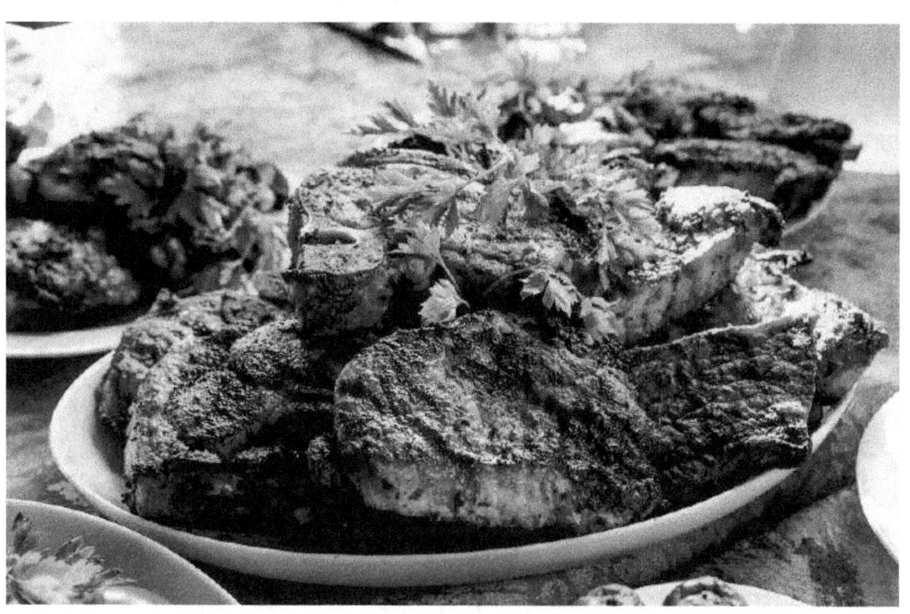

INGREDIENTS

-Lamb cubes
-cherry tomatoes
-red onions
-olive oil
-lemon juice
-cumin.

INSTRUCTIONS

1. Marinate lamb in olive oil, lemon juice, and cumin. Skewer with tomatoes and onions, grill until done.

NUTRITION INFO:

Fat: 35%, Protein: 60%, Carbs: 5%, Total Calories: ~180

6. Chicken and Vegetable Curry

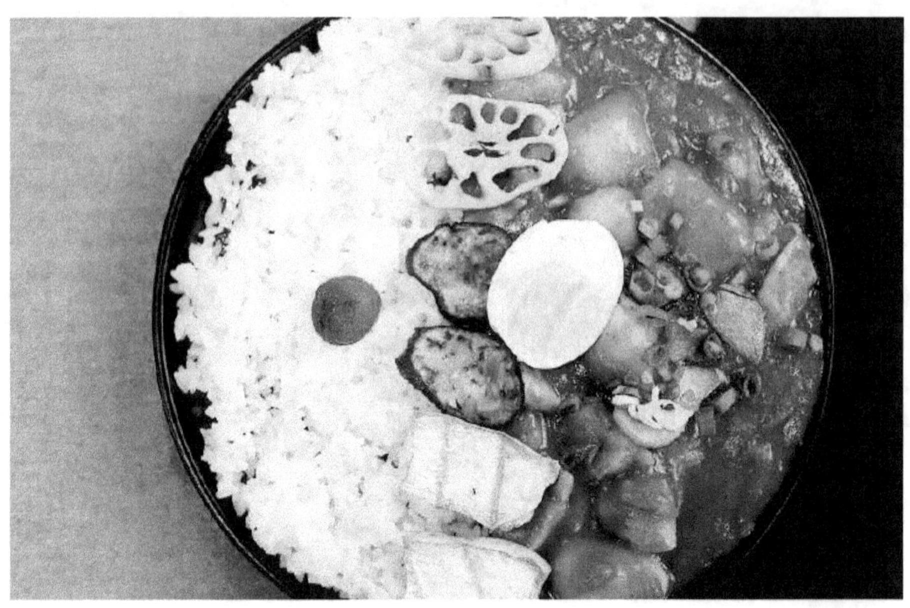

INGREDIENTS

-Chicken thighs

-mixed vegetables

-coconut milk

-curry paste

-turmeric.

INSTRUCTIONS

1. Cook chicken with vegetables, coconut milk, curry paste, and turmeric until tender.

NUTRITION INFO:

Fat: 30%, Protein: 40%, Carbs: 30%, Total Calories: ~220

7. Pork Loin with Rosemary Garlic Rub

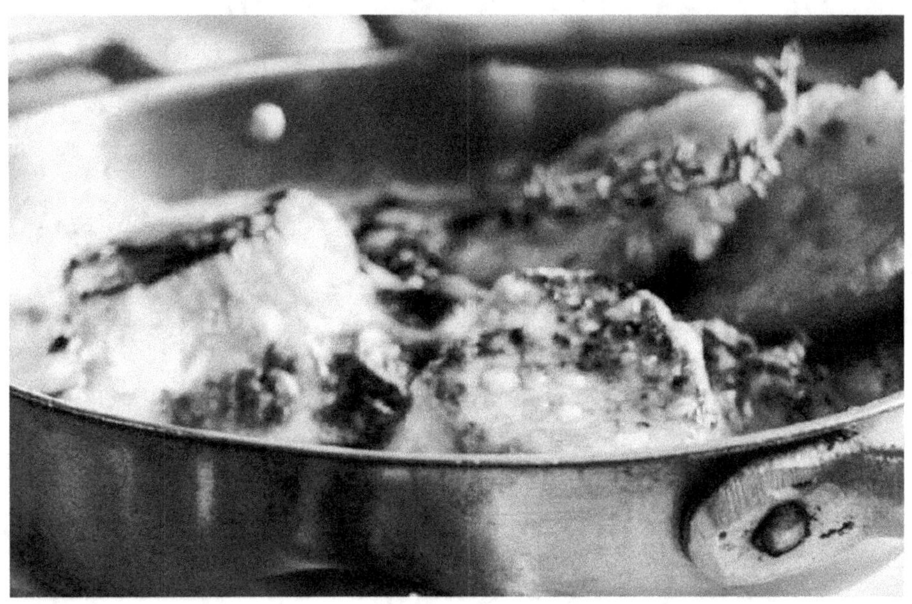

INGREDIENTS

- Pork loin
- rosemary
- garlic
- olive oil
- salt
- pepper.

INSTRUCTIONS

1. Rub pork with crushed garlic, rosemary, olive oil, salt, and pepper. Roast until cooked through.

NUTRITION INFO:

Fat: 20%, Protein: 55%, Carbs: 25%, Total Calories: ~170

8. Beef and Vegetable Soup

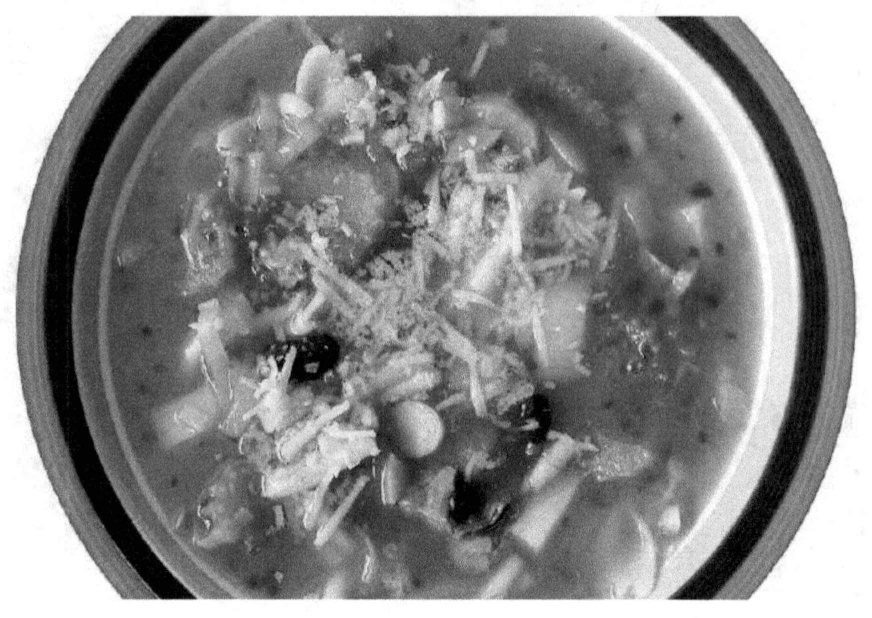

INGREDIENTS

- -Lean beef chunks
- -carrots
- -celery
- -onions
- -low-sodium beef broth
- -thyme.

INSTRUCTIONS

1. Simmer beef and vegetables in broth with thyme until beef is tender.

NUTRITION INFO:

Fat: 15%, Protein: 40%, Carbs: 45%, Total Calories: ~190

9. Chicken Lettuce Wraps

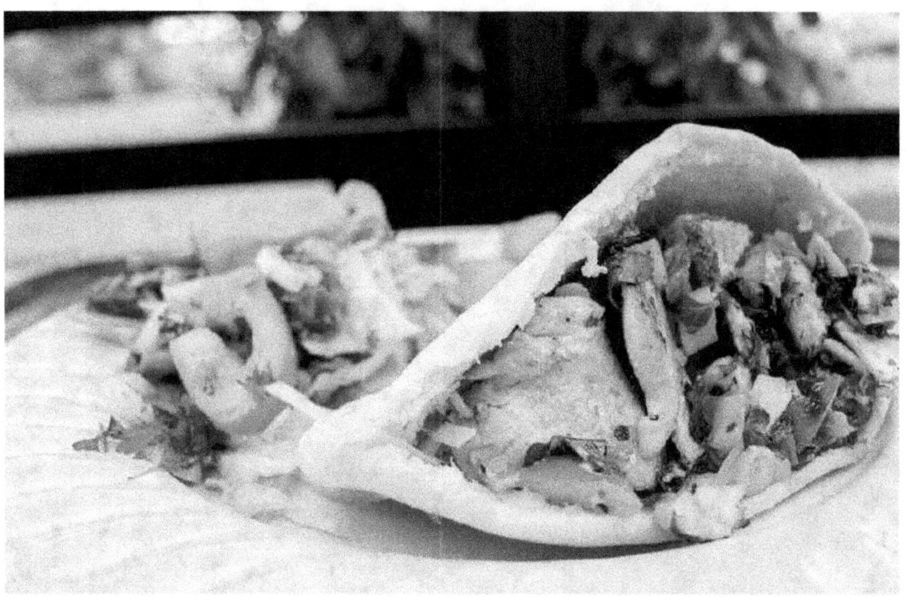

INGREDIENTS

-Ground chicken

-lettuce leaves

-mushrooms

-water chestnuts

-soy sauce

-ginger

-garlic.

INSTRUCTIONS

1. Cook chicken with mushrooms, water chestnuts, soy sauce, ginger, and garlic.
2. Serve in lettuce cups.

NUTRITION INFO:

Fat: 20%, Protein: 45%, Carbs: 35%, Total Calories: ~160

10. Pork and Broccoli Stir-Fry

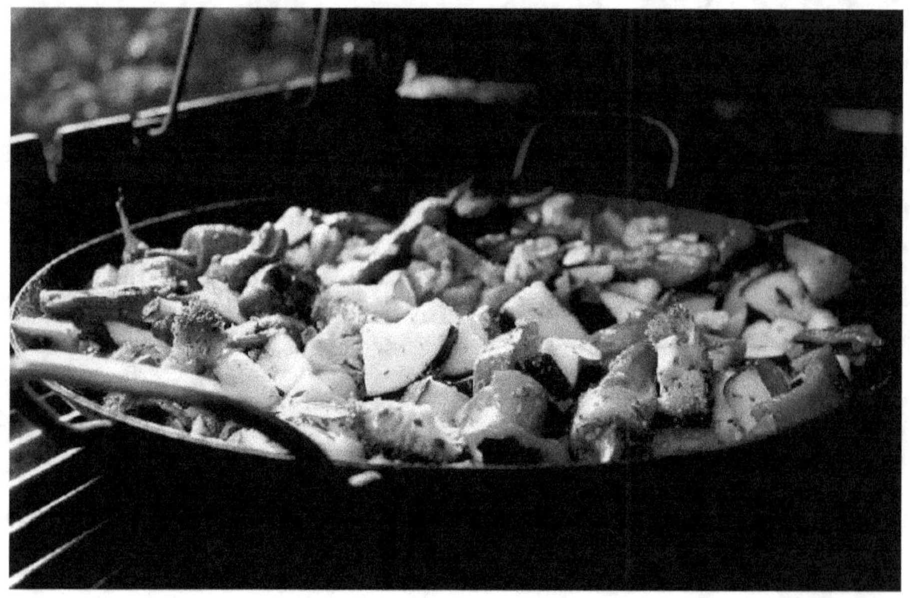

INGREDIENTS

-Pork tenderloin strips

-broccoli florets

-low-sodium soy sauce

-sesame oil

-honey

-garlic.

INSTRUCTIONS

1. Stir-fry pork and broccoli in sesame oil, soy sauce, honey, and garlic until cooked.

NUTRITION INFO:

Fat: 25%, Protein: 50%, Carbs: 25%, Total Calories: ~180

Legume and Bean
1. Lentil Soup

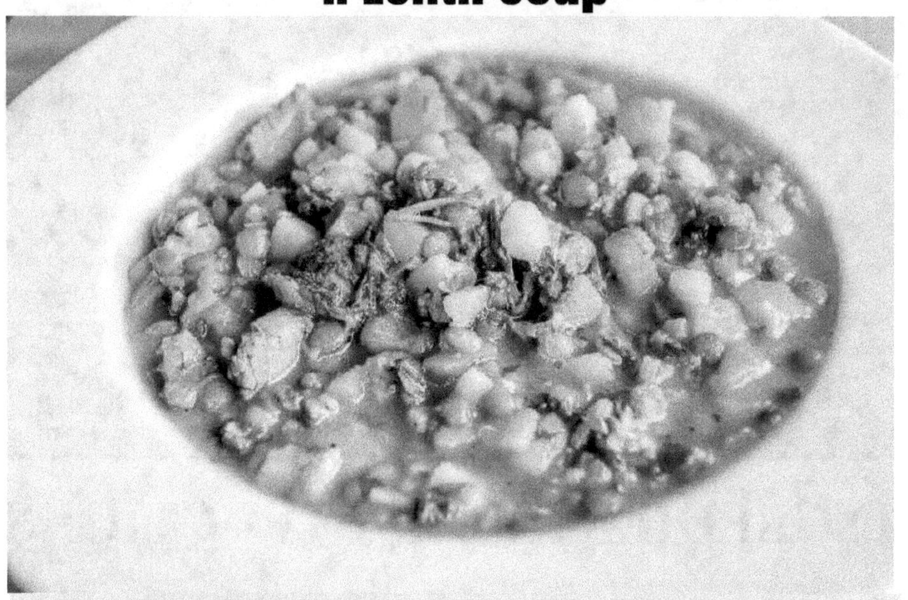

INGREDIENTS

- 1 cup dried lentils
- 4 cups vegetable or chicken broth
- 1 onion, chopped
- 2 carrots, diced
- 2 celery stalks, chopped
- 2 cloves garlic, minced
- 1 teaspoon cumin
- Salt and pepper to taste

INSTRUCTIONS

1. Rinse lentils and drain.

2. In a pot, sauté onions, carrots, and celery until softened. Add garlic and cook for 1-2 minutes.

3. Add lentils, broth, cumin, salt, and pepper. Bring to a boil, then simmer for 25-30 minutes until lentils are tender.

4. Adjust seasoning if needed. Serve hot.

NUTRITION INFO:

Fat: 5%, Protein: 30%, Carbs: 65%, Total Calories: ~180

2. Black Bean Salad

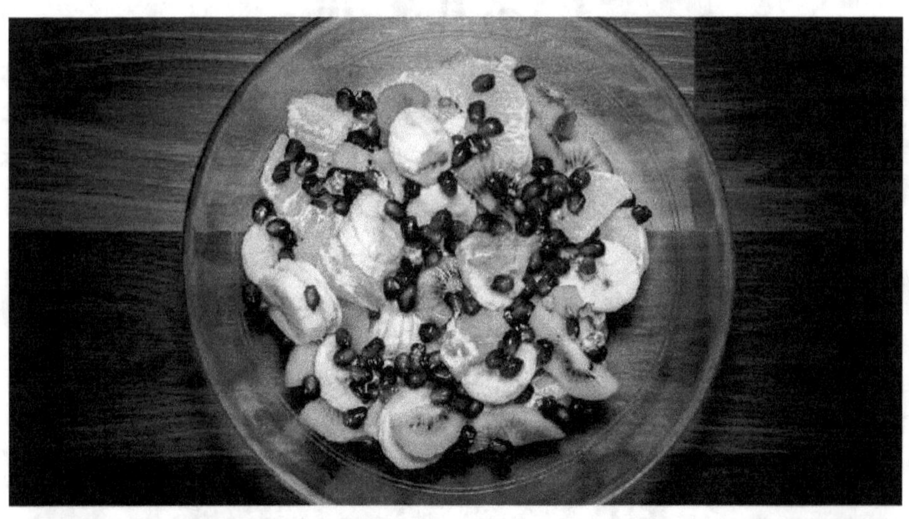

INGREDIENTS

- 2 cups cooked black beans
- 1 red bell pepper, diced
- 1 cup corn kernels (cooked or canned)
- 1/2 red onion, finely chopped
- 1 jalapeño, seeded and minced
- Fresh cilantro, chopped
- Lime juice, to taste
- Salt and pepper, to taste

INSTRUCTIONS

1. In a bowl, combine black beans, bell pepper, corn, red onion, jalapeño, and cilantro.

2. Drizzle lime juice, season with salt and pepper. Toss to combine.

3. Chill in the refrigerator for 30 minutes before serving.

NUTRITION INFO:

Fat: 5%, Protein: 25%, Carbs: 70%, Total Calories: ~160

3. Chickpea Curry

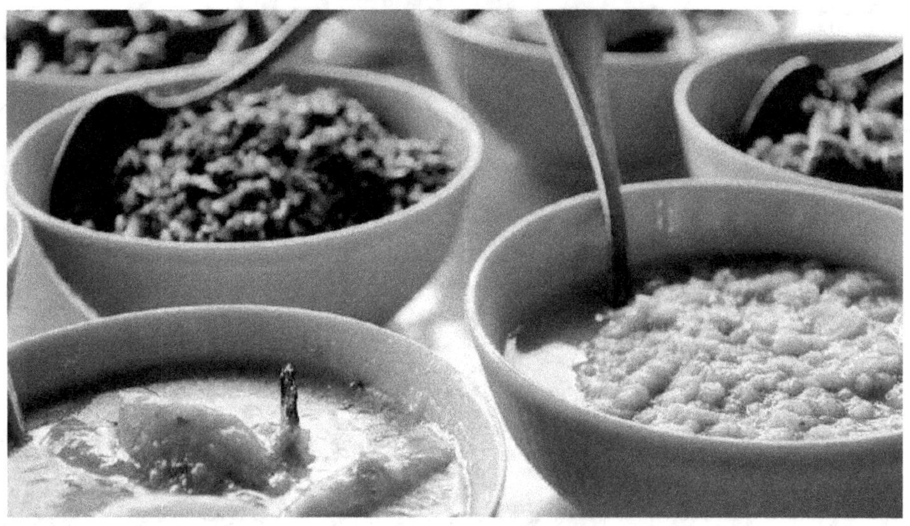

INGREDIENTS

- 2 cups cooked chickpeas
- 1 onion, finely chopped
- 2 cloves garlic, minced
- 1 can diced tomatoes
- 1 tablespoon curry powder
- 1 teaspoon turmeric
- 1 teaspoon ground cumin
- 1/2 teaspoon cayenne pepper (optional)
- Salt and pepper to taste
- Coconut milk (optional)

INSTRUCTIONS

1. Sauté onions and garlic until translucent. Add spices and cook for another minute.

2. Add diced tomatoes and chickpeas. Simmer for 15-20 minutes.

3. If desired, add coconut milk for creaminess. Season with salt and pepper.

4. Serve with naan bread or on top of rice.

NUTRITION INFO:

Fat: 10%, Protein: 20%, Carbs: 70%, Total Calories: ~200

4. Red Lentil Dahl

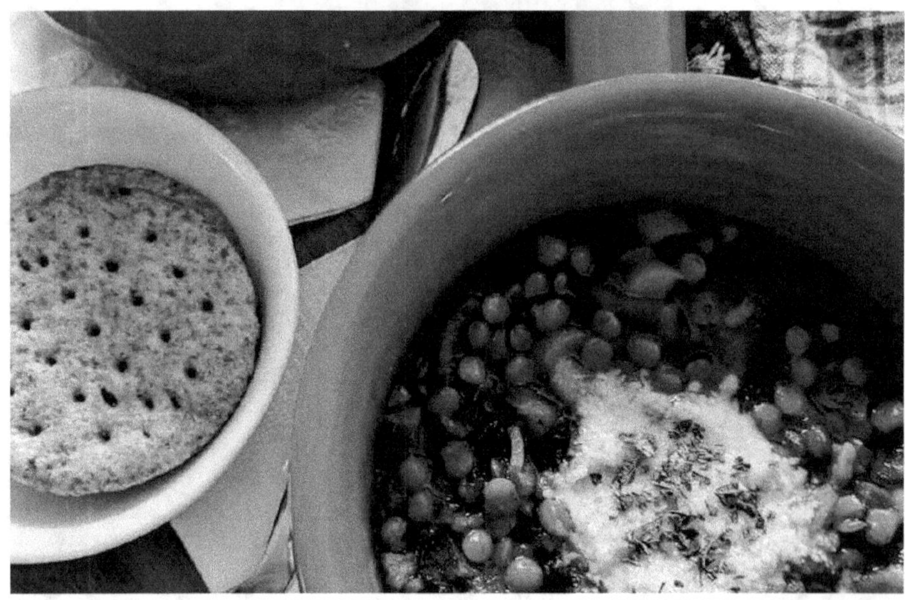

INGREDIENTS

- 1 cup red lentils
- 1 onion, chopped
- 2 cloves garlic, minced
- 1-inch piece of ginger, grated
- 1 can coconut milk
- 2 teaspoons curry powder
- 1 teaspoon turmeric
- 1 teaspoon ground cumin
- Fresh cilantro for garnish
- Salt and pepper to taste

INSTRUCTIONS

1. Sauté onion, garlic, and ginger until softened. Cook for one minute after adding the spices.

2. Add red lentils and coconut milk. Cook until the lentils are soft, about 20 to 25 minutes.

3. Season with salt and pepper. Garnish with fresh cilantro.

NUTRITION INFO:

Fat: 20%, Protein: 20%, Carbs: 60%, Total Calories: ~190

5. White Bean Soup

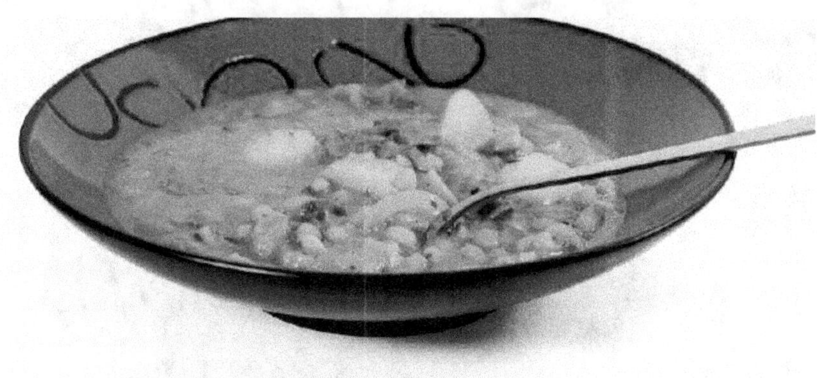

INGREDIENTS

- 2 cups cooked white beans (cannellini or navy)
- 4 cups vegetable or chicken broth
- 1 onion, chopped
- 2 carrots, diced
- 2 celery stalks, chopped
- 2 cloves garlic, minced
- Fresh rosemary and thyme
- Salt and pepper to taste

INSTRUCTIONS

1. Sauté onions, carrots, and celery until softened. Add garlic and cook for 1-2 minutes.

2. Add white beans, broth, fresh herbs, salt, and pepper. Simmer for 20-25 minutes.

3. Mash some of the beans to thicken the soup if desired. Adjust seasoning and serve hot.

NUTRITION INFO:

Fat: 5%, Protein: 25%, Carbs: 70%, Total Calories: ~170

6. Three Bean Salad

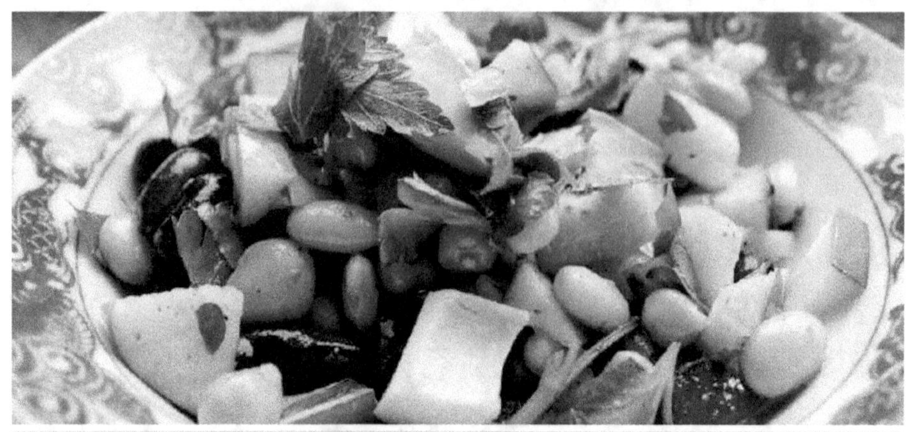

INGREDIENTS

- 1 can kidney beans, drained and rinsed
- 1 can black beans, drained and rinsed
- 1 can chickpeas, drained and rinsed
- 1 red onion, finely chopped
- 1 red bell pepper, diced
- Fresh parsley, chopped
- ¼ cup olive oil
- 2 tablespoons apple cider vinegar
- Salt and pepper to taste

INSTRUCTIONS

1. In a large bowl, combine all the beans, red onion, bell pepper, and parsley.

2. In a small bowl, whisk together olive oil, apple cider vinegar, salt, and pepper.

3. Pour the dressing over the bean mixture and toss until well coated.

4. Refrigerate for at least 30 minutes before serving.

NUTRITION INFO:

Fat: 25%, Protein: 30%, Carbs: 45%, Total Calories: ~180

7. Black-Eyed Pea Stew

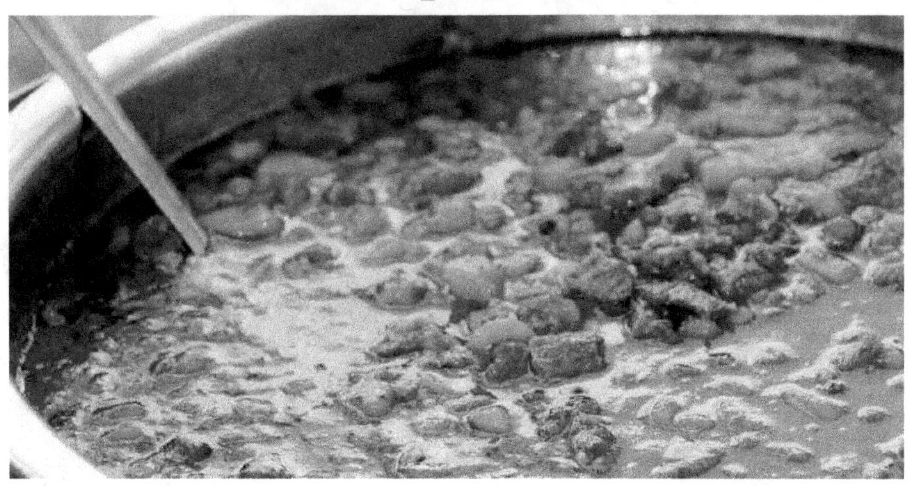

INGREDIENTS

- 2 cups of rinsed and soaked black-eyed peas
- 1 onion, chopped
- 3 garlic cloves, minced
- 2 tomatoes, diced
- 2 cups vegetable broth
- 1 teaspoon paprika
- ½ teaspoon cayenne pepper (optional)
- Fresh parsley for garnish
- Salt and pepper to taste

INSTRUCTIONS

1. Sauté garlic and onions in a pot until they become translucent.

2. Add soaked black-eyed peas, tomatoes, vegetable broth, paprika, and cayenne pepper. Simmer for 40-45 minutes until peas are tender.

3. Season with salt and pepper. Garnish with fresh parsley before serving.

NUTRITION INFO:

Fat: 5%, Protein: 20%, Carbs: 75%, Total Calories: ~160

8. Split Pea Soup

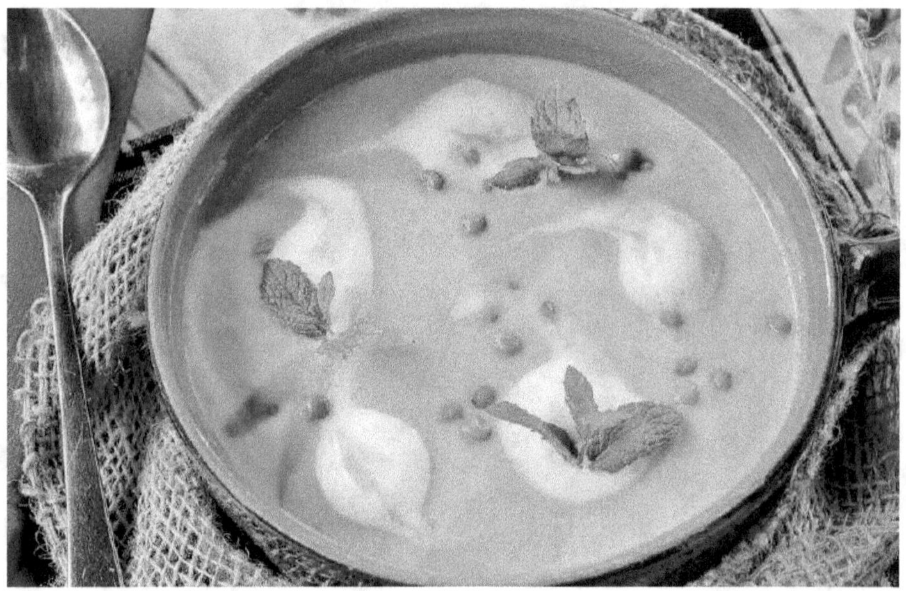

INGREDIENTS

- 1 cup dried split peas
- 1 onion, chopped
- 2 carrots, diced
- 2 celery stalks, chopped
- 2 cloves garlic, minced
- 4 cups vegetable or chicken broth
- 1 bay leaf
- Fresh thyme
- Salt and pepper to taste

INSTRUCTIONS

1. Rinse split peas and drain.
2. In a pot, sauté onions, carrots, celery, and garlic until softened.
3. Add split peas, broth, bay leaf, and thyme. Simmer for 45-50 minutes until the peas are tender.
4. Remove bay leaf, season with salt

NUTRITION INFO:

Fat: 5%, Protein: 25%, Carbs: 70%, Total Calories: ~170

9. Pinto Bean Tacos

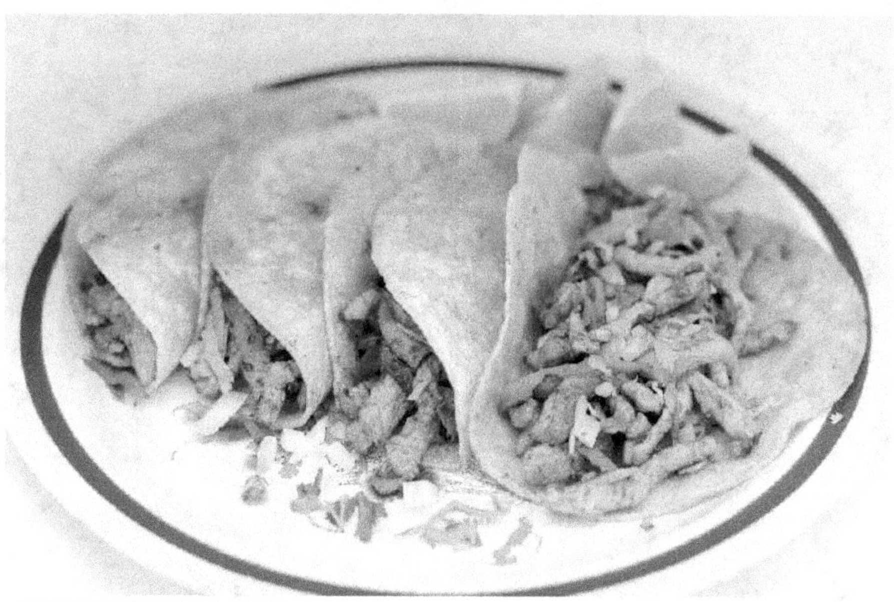

INGREDIENTS

- 2 cups cooked pinto beans
- 1 onion, diced
- 2 cloves garlic, minced
- 1 teaspoon chili powder
- ½ teaspoon cumin
- ½ teaspoon paprika
- Corn tortillas
- Toppings: diced tomatoes, shredded lettuce, avocado, salsa

INSTRUCTIONS

1. Sauté onions and garlic until golden. Add cooked pinto beans and spices, cook for 5-7 minutes.

2. Warm corn tortillas. Fill with the bean mixture and desired toppings.

3. Serve immediately.

NUTRITION INFO:

Fat: 5%, Protein: 20%, Carbs: 75%, Total Calories: ~160

10. Creamy Bean and Kale Soup

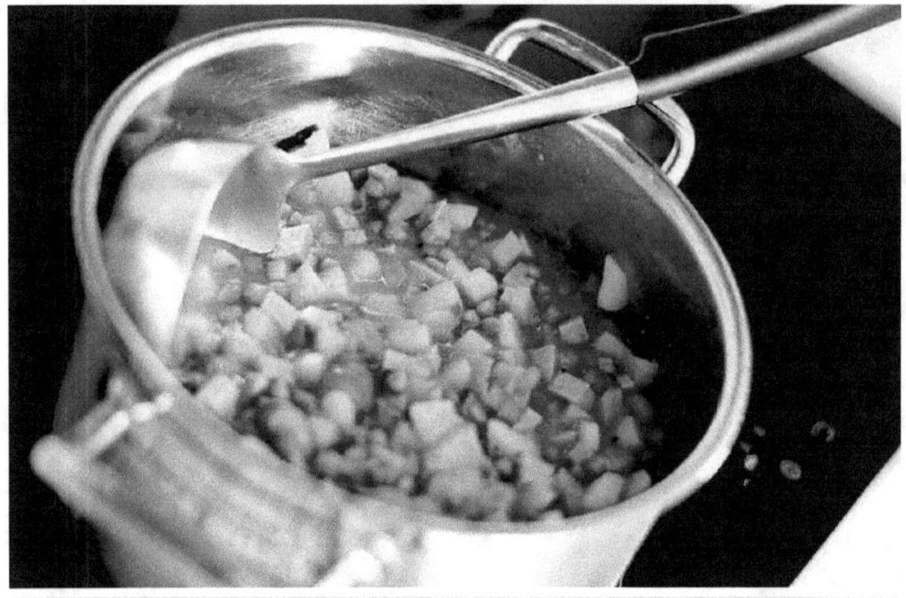

INGREDIENTS

- 2 cups cooked navy beans
- 1 onion, chopped
- 2 carrots, diced
- 2 celery stalks, chopped
- 2 cloves garlic, minced
- 4 cups vegetable broth
- 2 cups chopped kale
- Fresh rosemary
- Salt and pepper to taste

INSTRUCTIONS

1. Sauté onions, carrots, celery, and garlic until tender.

2. Add cooked navy beans, vegetable broth, kale, and rosemary. Simmer for 15-20 minutes.

3. Season with salt and pepper. Serve hot.

NUTRITION INFO:

Fat: 5%, Protein: 25%, Carbs: 70%, Total Calories: ~180

Beverage
1. Green Tea

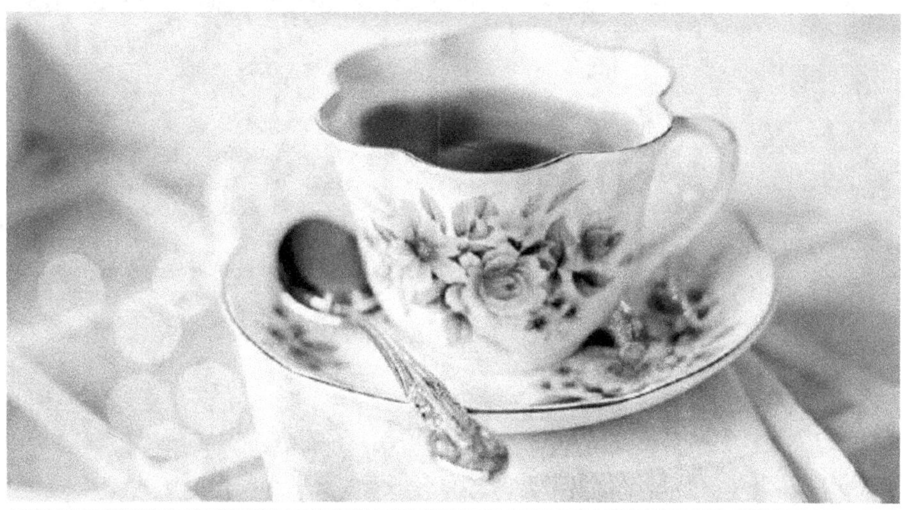

INGREDIENTS

- Green tea leaves or tea bags
- Hot water

INSTRUCTIONS

1. Steep green tea leaves or tea bags in hot water for 3-5 minutes.
2. Strain and enjoy.

NUTRITION INFO:

No fat, no protein, no carbs, Total Calories: ~0

3. Sparkling Water with Lemon

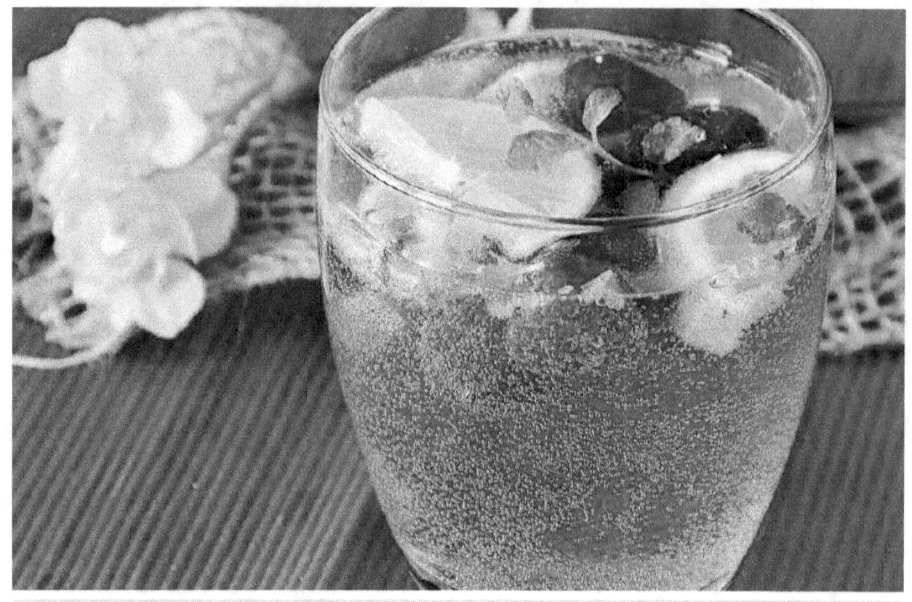

INGREDIENTS

- Sparkling water
- Fresh lemon juice
- Optional: Stevia or other low-calorie sweetener

INSTRUCTIONS

1. Mix sparkling water with fresh lemon juice.

2. Add sweetener if desired, stir well, and serve over ice.

NUTRITION INFO:

No fat, no protein, minimal carbs, Total Calories: ~5

5. Almond Milk Latte

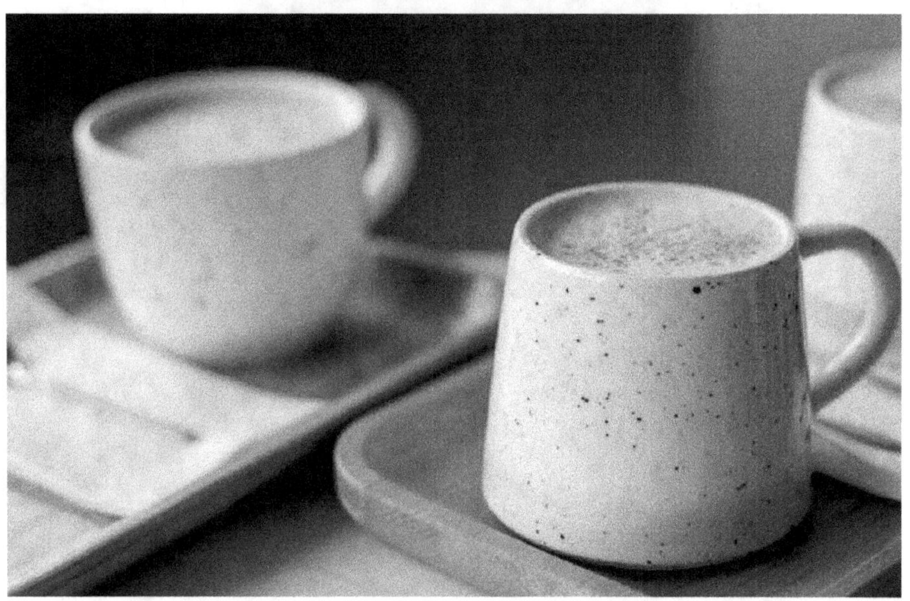

INGREDIENTS

- 1 cup unsweetened almond milk
- 1 shot of espresso or strong brewed coffee

INSTRUCTIONS

1. Heat almond milk on the stovetop or microwave until hot.
2. Froth the milk if desired. Pour over the espresso or coffee.

NUTRITION INFO:

Fat: 30%, Protein: 15%, Carbs: 55%, Total Calories: ~40-50

6. Golden Milk (Turmeric Milk)

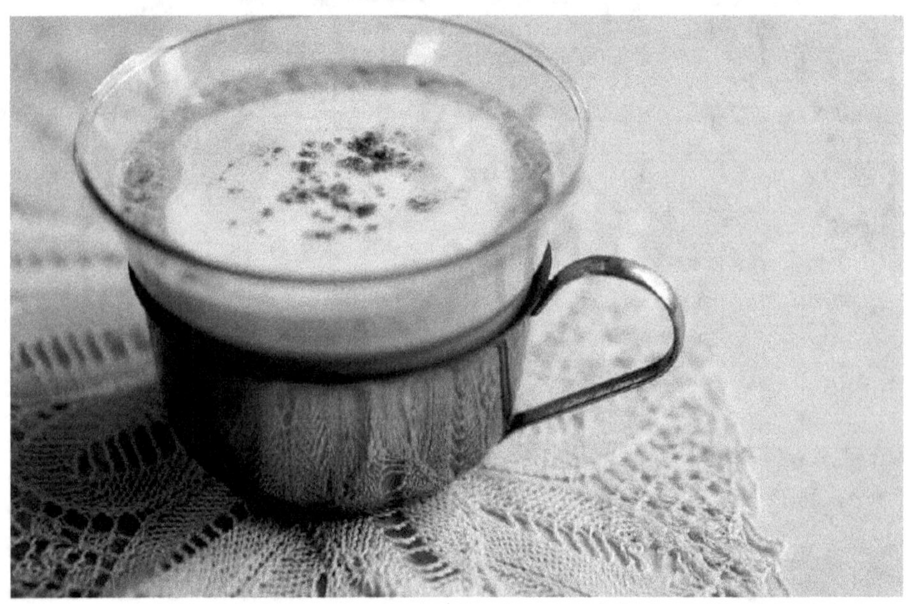

INGREDIENTS

- 1 cup unsweetened almond milk
- ½ teaspoon ground turmeric
- ½ teaspoon ground cinnamon
- Pinch of black pepper
- Optional: Sweetener like honey or stevia

INSTRUCTIONS

1. Warm almond milk on the stovetop.
2. Whisk in turmeric, cinnamon, black pepper, and sweetener if desired. Heat until steaming.

NUTRITION INFO:

Fat: 20%, Protein: 10%, Carbs: 70%, Total Calories: ~50

7. Berry Smoothie

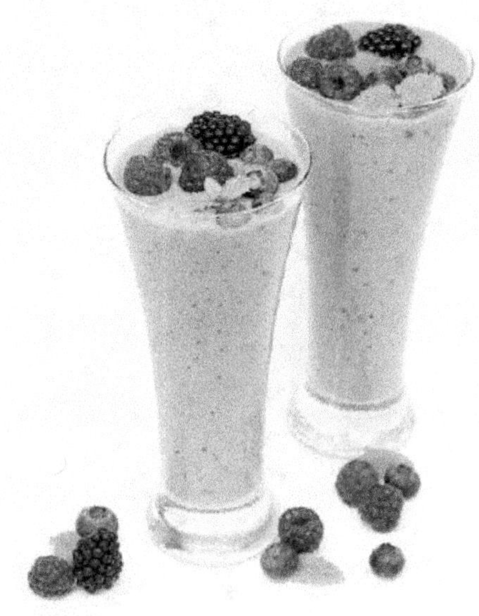

INGREDIENTS

- 1 cup mixed berries (fresh or frozen)
- 1 cup unsweetened almond milk
- ½ banana
- One tablespoon chia or flax seeds, optional

INSTRUCTIONS

1. Blend all ingredients until smooth.

NUTRITION INFO:

Fat: 15%, Protein: 10%, Carbs: 75%, Total Calories: ~80

8. Coconut Water

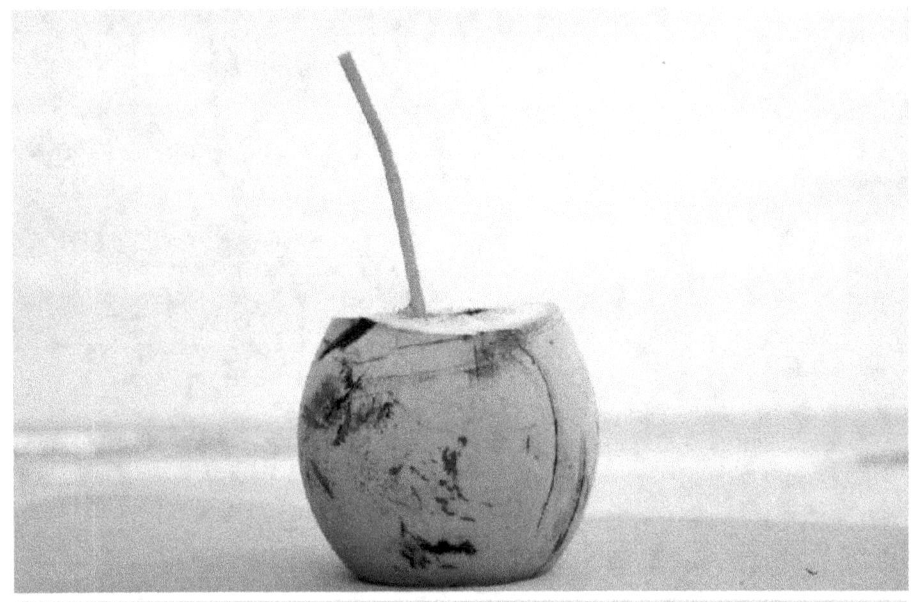

INGREDIENTS

- Coconut water (fresh or bottled)

INSTRUCTIONS

1. Simply serve coconut water chilled.

NUTRITION INFO:

No fat, no protein, minimal carbs, Total Calories: ~45

9. Herbal Infusion with Ginger and Lemon

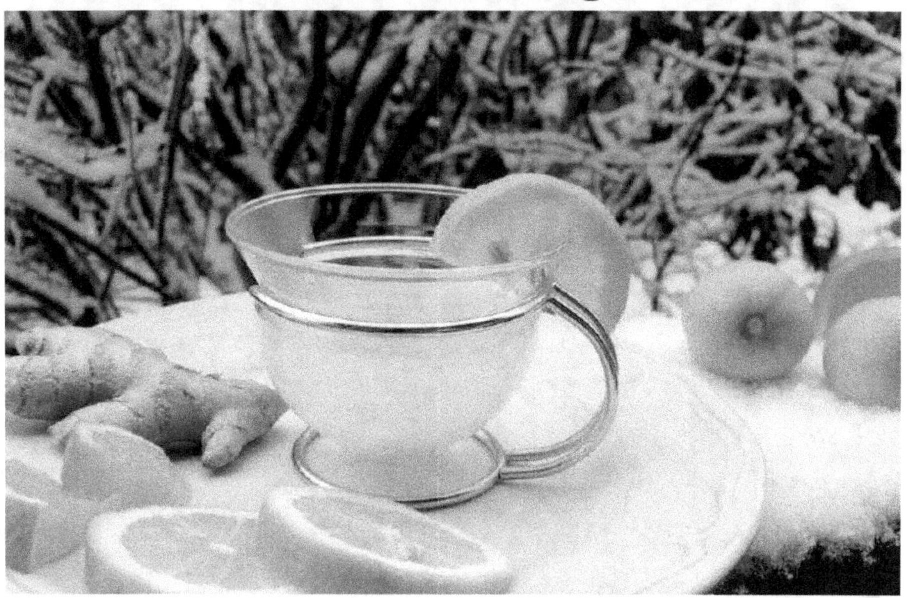

INGREDIENTS

- Fresh ginger slices
- Lemon slices
- Herbal tea bag (chamomile, peppermint, etc.)
- Hot water

INSTRUCTIONS

1. Steep ginger, lemon, and herbal tea bag in hot water for 3-5 minutes.
2. Strain and enjoy.

NUTRITION INFO:

No fat, no protein, minimal carbs, Total Calories: ~0

10. Tomato Juice

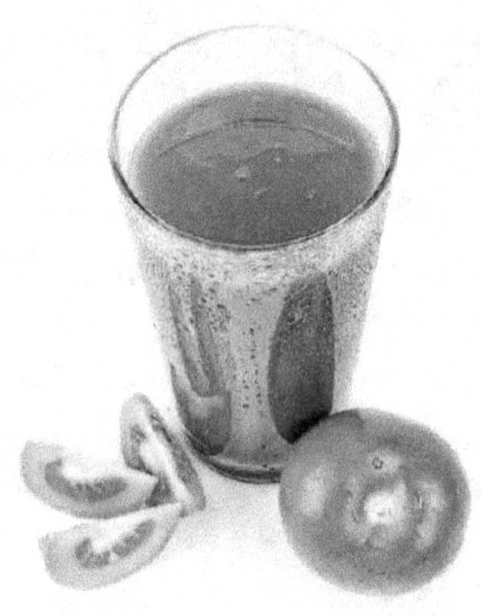

INGREDIENTS

- Fresh tomatoes or low-sodium tomato juice

INSTRUCTIONS

1. Juice fresh tomatoes or use store-bought low-sodium tomato juice.

NUTRITION INFO:

Fat: 5%, Protein: 15%, Carbs: 80%, Total Calories: ~50

Condiments, oils, and sauces
1. Homemade Pesto Sauce

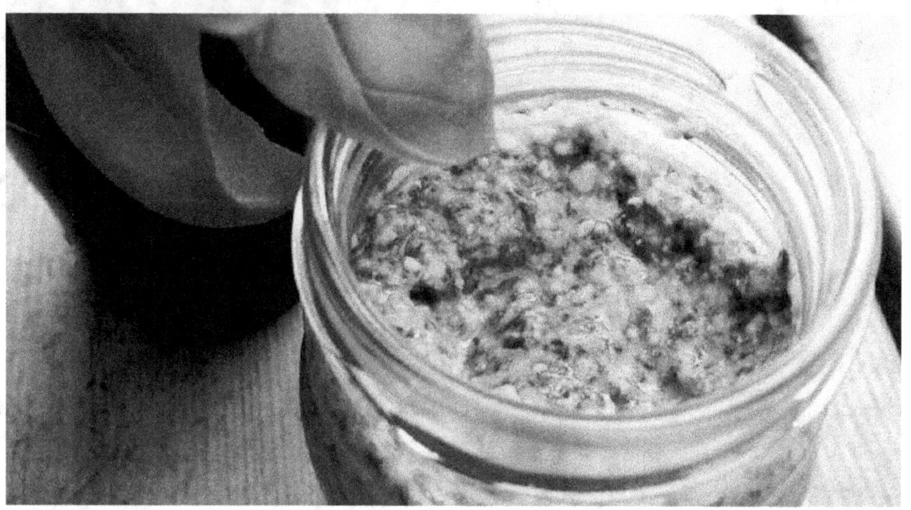

INGREDIENTS

- 2 cups fresh basil leaves
- 1/2 cup grated Parmesan cheese
- half a cup of walnuts or pine nuts
- 2 garlic cloves
- 1/2 cup extra virgin olive oil
- Salt and pepper to taste

INSTRUCTIONS

1. Blend basil, Parmesan, pine nuts, and garlic in a food processor until finely chopped.
2. While blending, gradually add olive oil until the mixture forms a smooth paste.
3. Season with salt and pepper. Adjust consistency and taste as desired.

NUTRITION INFO:

Fat: 90%, Protein: 5%, Carbs: 5%, Total Calories: ~80

2. Guacamole

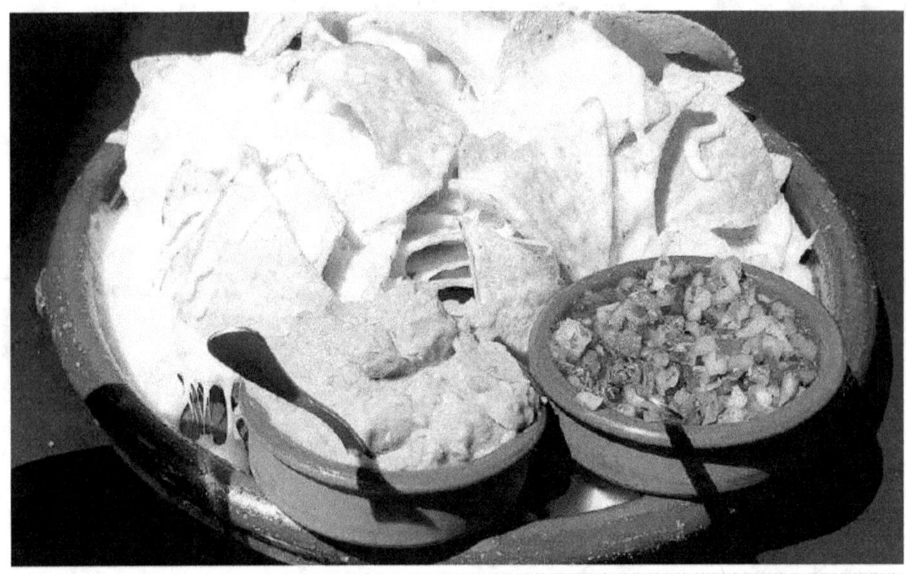

INGREDIENTS

- 2 ripe avocados
- 1 tomato, diced
- 1/4 cup red onion, finely chopped
- 1/4 cup cilantro, chopped
- 1 lime, juiced
- Salt and pepper to taste

INSTRUCTIONS

1. Mash avocados in a bowl.
2. Stir in diced tomato, red onion, cilantro, lime juice, salt, and pepper.
3. Mix until well combined.

NUTRITION INFO:

Fat: 90%, Protein: 5%, Carbs: 5%, Total Calories: ~50

3. Homemade Tomato Sauce

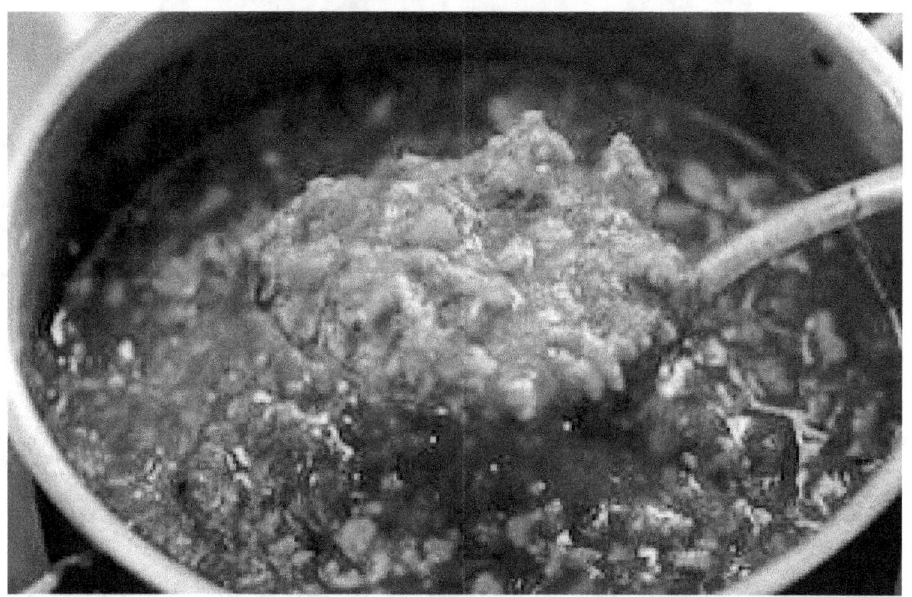

INGREDIENTS

- 6 ripe tomatoes, diced
- 2 garlic cloves, minced
- 1 onion, finely chopped
- 2 tablespoons olive oil
- 1 teaspoon dried oregano
- Salt and pepper to taste

INSTRUCTIONS

1. Heat olive oil in a pan. Add minced garlic and chopped onion. Sauté until translucent.

2. Add diced tomatoes and dried oregano. Cook until the sauce thickens, about 20 to 30 minutes.

3. Season with salt and pepper. Blend for a smoother consistency if desired.

NUTRITION INFO:

Fat: 80%, Protein: 5%, Carbs: 15%, Total Calories: ~40

4. Tahini Sauce

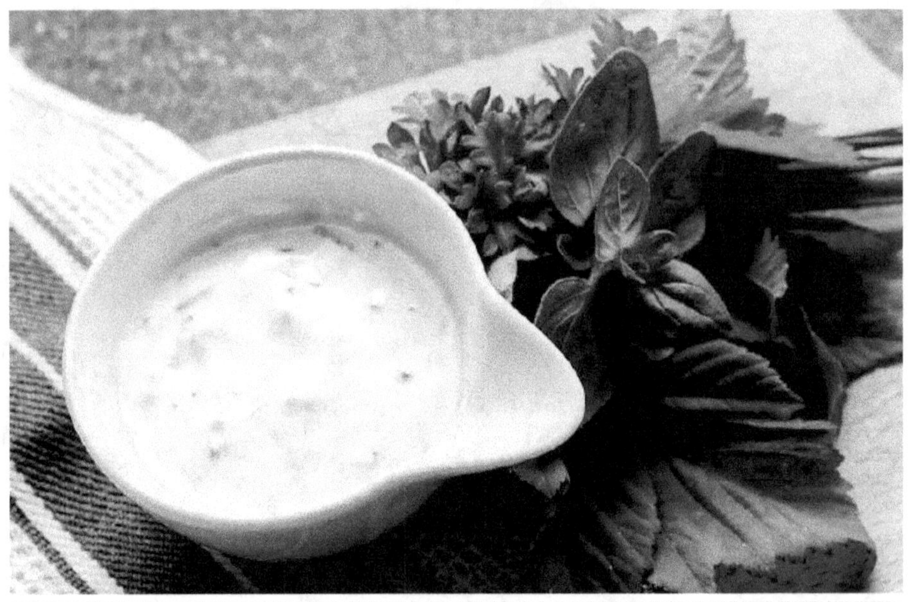

INGREDIENTS

- -1/2 cup tahini
- -2 tablespoons lemon juice
- -2 garlic cloves, minced
- -1/4 cup water (or more for desired consistency)
- -Salt to taste

INSTRUCTIONS

1. Whisk together tahini, lemon juice, minced garlic, and water until smooth.
2. Stir in additional water if the consistency seems too thick.
3. Season with salt to taste.

NUTRITION INFO:

Fat: 80%, Protein: 10%, Carbs: 10%, Total Calories: ~50

5. Sugar-Free BBQ Sauce

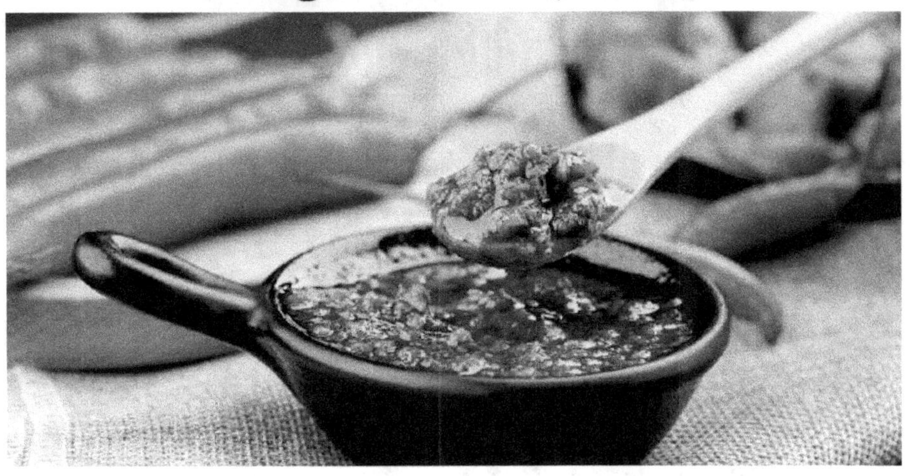

INGREDIENTS

-1 cup tomato sauce (no sugar added)

-2 tablespoons apple cider vinegar

-1 tablespoon Worcestershire sauce (look for sugar-free)

-1 tablespoon Dijon mustard

-1 teaspoon smoked paprika

-1 teaspoon garlic powder

-1/2 teaspoon onion powder

-1/4 teaspoon cayenne pepper (optional)

-Salt and pepper to taste

INSTRUCTIONS

1. Combine all ingredients in a saucepan.

2. For ten to fifteen minutes, simmer over low heat, stirring from time to time.

3. Allow to cool before utilizing it as a marinade or sauce.

NUTRITION INFO:

Fat: 5%, Protein: 5%, Carbs: 90%, Total Calories: ~15

Dairy and soy alternative
1. Almond Milk Chia Pudding

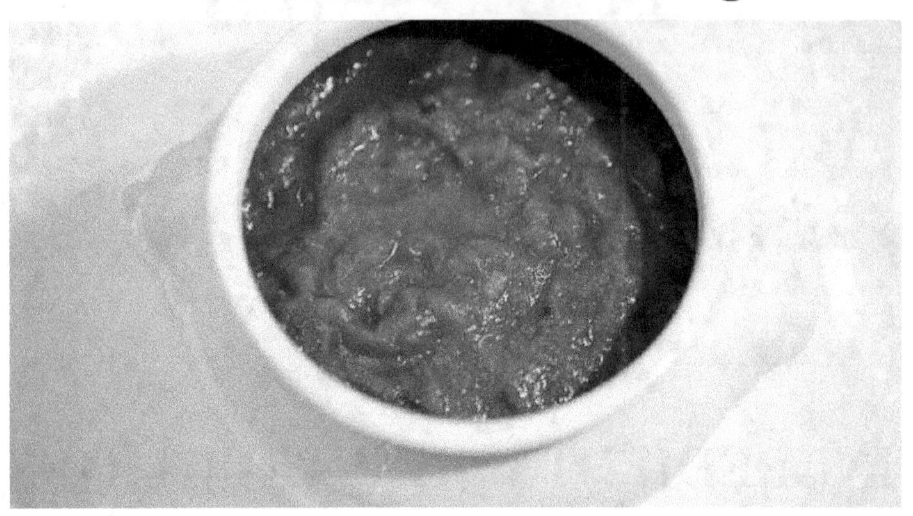

INGREDIENTS

- 1 cup unsweetened almond milk
- 1/4 cup chia seeds
- One tablespoon of maple syrup or your preferred sweetener
- 1/2 teaspoon vanilla extract
- Topping options include sliced almonds and fresh berries.

INSTRUCTIONS

1. Mix almond milk, chia seeds, maple syrup, and vanilla extract in a bowl.

2. Refrigerate for at least 2 hours or overnight, stirring occasionally until thickened.

3. Serve topped with fresh berries and sliced almonds if desired.

NUTRITION INFO:

Fat: 50%, Protein: 10%, Carbs: 40%, Total Calories: ~150

2. Tofu Scramble

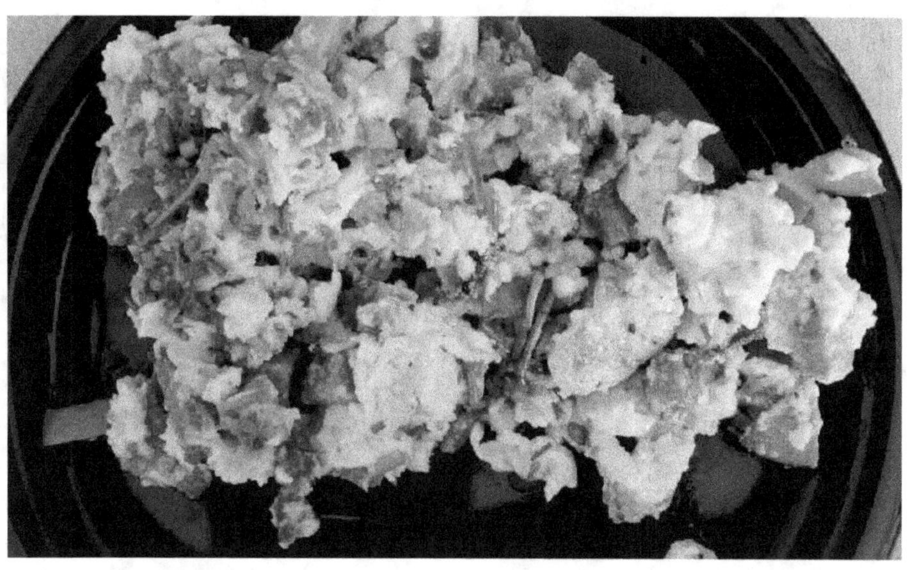

INGREDIENTS

- 1 block firm tofu, crumbled
- 1 tablespoon olive oil
- 1/2 onion, diced
- 1 bell pepper, diced
- 1 teaspoon turmeric
- Salt and pepper to taste
- Optional: spinach, nutritional yeast

INSTRUCTIONS

1. Heat olive oil in a pan, add diced onion and bell pepper. Sauté until softened.
2. Add crumbled tofu, turmeric, salt, and pepper. Bring to a boil and cook for 5 to 7 minutes.
3. Optional: Add spinach and nutritional yeast for extra flavor.
4. Serve warm.

NUTRITION INFO:

Fat: 45%, Protein: 35%, Carbs: 20%, Total Calories: ~180

3. Coconut Milk Curry

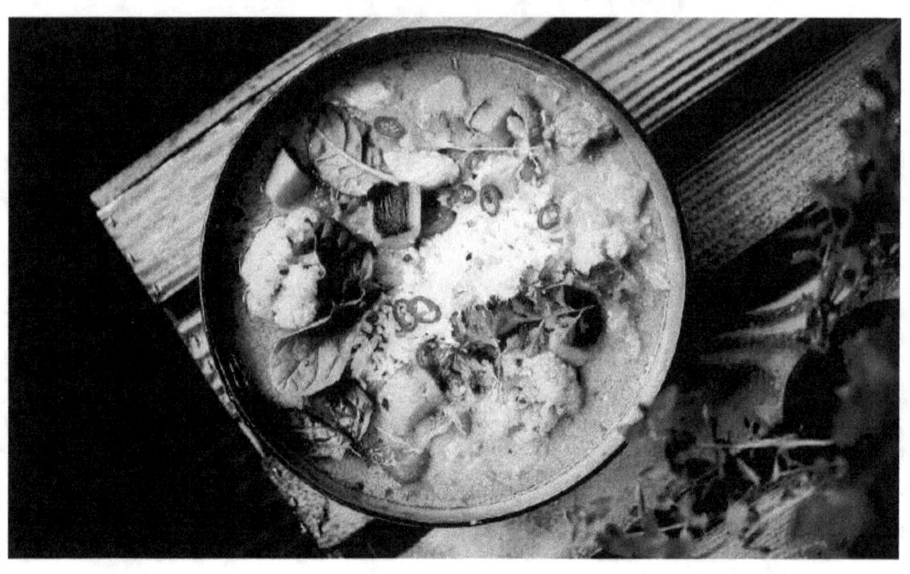

INGREDIENTS

- 1 can coconut milk
- 2 tablespoons red curry paste
- Variety of vegetables (carrots, broccoli, and bell peppers)
- Tofu or chickpeas for protein
- Salt and pepper to taste
- Optional: cilantro for garnish

INSTRUCTIONS

1. In a pan, heat coconut milk and red curry paste. Stir until combined.
2. Add assorted vegetables and protein of choice. Simmer until the veggies are tender.
3. Season with salt and pepper. Garnish with cilantro.
4. Serve over rice or quinoa.

NUTRITION INFO:

Fat: 60%, Protein: 15%, Carbs: 25%, Total Calories: ~220

4. Soy Yogurt Parfait

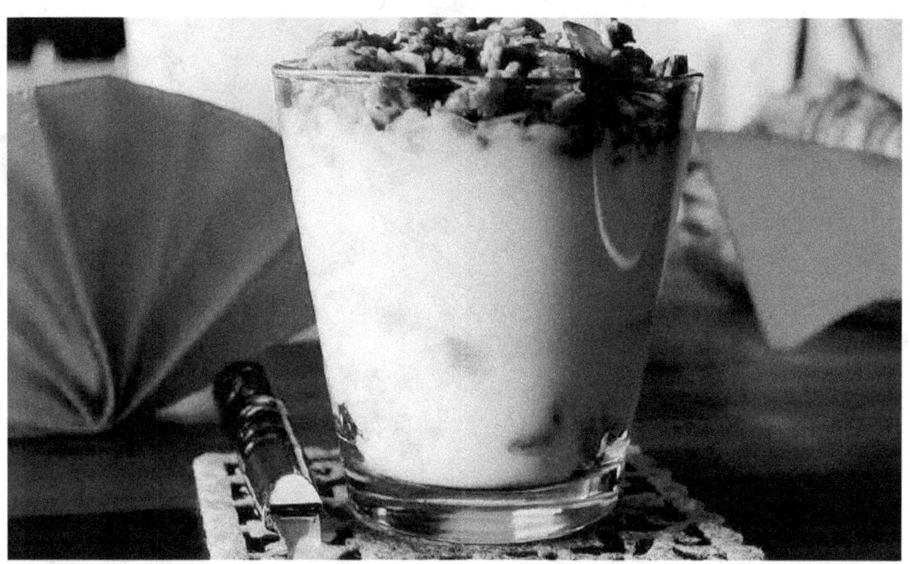

INGREDIENTS

- 1 cup soy yogurt
- 1/2 cup mixed berries
- 2 tablespoons granola
- 1 tablespoon honey or sweetener of choice (optional)

INSTRUCTIONS

1. In a glass, layer soy yogurt, mixed berries, and granola.
2. If you would like, drizzle with honey or sweetener.
3. Repeat layers and serve chilled.

NUTRITION INFO:

Fat: 20%, Protein: 15%, Carbs: 65%, Total Calories: ~120

5. Oat Milk Pancakes

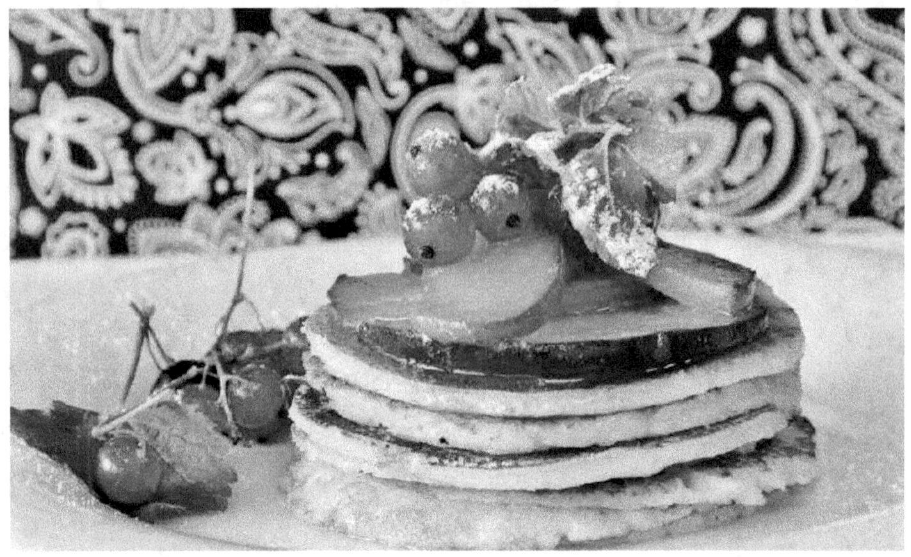

INGREDIENTS

- 1 cup oat milk
- 1 cup oat flour
- 1 tablespoon maple syrup
- 1 teaspoon baking powder
- Pinch of salt
- Coconut oil for cooking

INSTRUCTIONS

1. In a bowl, mix oat milk, oat flour, maple syrup, baking powder, and salt until smooth.

2. Heat coconut oil in a pan. To prepare pancakes, pour the batter onto the pan.

3. Cook until bubbles form, then flip and cook the other side.

4. Serve with fruit or toppings of choice.

NUTRITION INFO:

Fat: 30%, Protein: 15%, Carbs: 55%, Total Calories: ~180